This book is due for return on or before the last date shown below.

About the Author

John McKenna has a science degree and a medical degree and has been practising nutritional medicine for over 25 years. He has come out of retirement to set up The Food Clinic which deals with weight loss issues. He is the bestselling author of *Hard to Stomach*, *Natural Alternatives to Antibiotics*, *Alternatives to Tranquillisers* and *The Big Fat Secret*. His books have been translated into most European languages.

Good Food

Can You Trust What You Are Eating?

John McKenna BA, MB, ChB

Gill & Macmillan

Gill & Macmillan
Hume Avenue, Park West, Dublin 12
www.gillmacmillanbooks.ie

© John McKenna 2013
978 07171 5425 8

Index compiled by Eileen O'Neill
Illustrations by Derry Dillon
Typography design by Make Communication
Print origination by Carole Lynch
Printed and bound by SPRINT-print Ltd., Ireland

This book is typeset in Linotype Minion and Neue Helvetica.

The paper used in this book comes from the wood pulp of
managed forests. For every tree felled, at least one tree is
planted, thereby renewing natural resources.

A CIP catalogue record for this book is available
from the British Library.

5 4 3 2

Contents

*I wish to dedicate this book to my mother,
Kathleen McKenna, for the high standards
that she lived by, especially in the selection
and preparation of food. She was a wonderful
mother whose love was boundless. She dedicated
her life to caring for her children and so I in
turn dedicate this book to her as a mark of
respect and as repayment for all the wonderful
things she did for me while growing up. I love you
very much and wait to be reunited in spirit.*

Acknowledgements

I would firstly like to thank my editor, Fergal Tobin, for agreeing to publish this book and for his help during the writing of it. I would also like to thank the Price-Pottenger Nutrition Foundation for allowing me to use a story in Dr Price's book *Nutrition and Physical Degeneration*. I would also like to thank a local farmer, Aidan O'Connor, for his help with all my questions. A big thanks to my good friend Dr Pradeep Chadha for all his kindness and encouragement during the writing of this. I would also like to thank him for his collaboration in my first e-book, *The Big Fat Secret*. A big thanks to Jaqui Lyons for her kindness and encouragement as well. I sincerely hope your health improves as you are needed and loved by many. Also, big thanks to my children for their help and support during the past few years. I love you all very much. A massive thank you to all my patients, who have been so kind and supportive of me over the years. Your kindness and support are appreciated very much, especially in the last few years. I have learned so much from you and have been privileged to have met you all. Finally, a special thank you to my mother, Kathleen, who is in spirit form now but who dedicated her life to looking after her children and to providing the best food she could source. Her brilliant work has been a major influence in my life and especially in the writing of this book. I have therefore decided to dedicate the book to her, as she was such a special person.

Introduction

I have rewritten this manuscript five times. Initially I just wanted to shed some light and convey some common sense on what has become the single most important issue affecting people in the Western world. In effect, I wanted to contrast my diet growing up in Northern Ireland and my diet during the years I spent in different parts of Africa with the diet of people living in Europe today. The Western diet has undergone a revolution in the space of a few decades.

Then I realised I had to address other issues, such as the way people are informed about nutrition. I also had to deal with the food pyramid, which is the main tool used by schools, universities and governments to educate the population about good dietary habits. In dealing with the topic of the food pyramid I was obliged to deal with the thorny issue of animal or saturated fat in the diet and the even thornier issue of sugar. Dealing with the reduction of animal fats in foods and the replacement of this fat with sugar led to a lot of political intrigue.

This unfortunately led to the unearthing of serious events that took place in the United States during the 1970s that now threaten the health of almost every nation that consumes processed foodstuffs. I not only had to research the negative role of food manufacturers in shaping the diet of modern people all over the world, I also had to examine the effects of the chemical industry on farming, which has undergone a revolution in my lifetime. This led to looking at the issue of natural pastures versus unnatural pastures as well as the issue of soil as the link between all living creatures and the planet we occupy. This in turn led to ecological and philosophical issues that drive our society. Each draft has attempted to dig a bit deeper into the issue of food and how it affects all of us.

However, despite all the negative effects we humans have had on the world we live in, I wanted to describe some of the magical events that make life possible and make good food possible for you and your family. I have witnessed this magic first hand growing up in Northern Ireland and working in Africa. Writing these various scripts has given me some insight into my own life. I now better understand why I had to grow up in the heart of the countryside to appreciate simplicity, especially simple foods. I also understand why I spent so many years living and working in Africa, where I was able to see how more isolated people lived and what foods they ate. This African experience provided a powerful contrast to my Western way of eating and living.

Writing this book has also helped me realise my deep interest in all things nutritional. For most of my clinical practice I've used diet and nutritional supplements to treat a range of medical conditions. In rural Africa, diseases of the Western world such as heart disease, arthritis, diabetes, etc. don't exist. However, once these rural people enter urban areas and start abandoning their traditional diet in favour of a more Western diet, all these Western disorders begin to manifest. Reversing these diseases, including many forms of cancer, is possible simply by altering their diet – amazing but true. The chapter devoted to Dr Weston Price's research is powerful testimony to this fact (see Chapter 2).

The real message that I wanted to convey in this final draft of the book is a little deeper than that. It's a message of self-reliance. Don't expect society to change to suit your opinions or needs. It's time to become less reliant on the structures in your society and more reliant on your own ability. The power lies with you. There are vested interests at work trying to control you, your government and all the structures designed to protect you, such as the Food Safety Authority (the Food and Drug Administration in the us), national associations such as your national heart association, professional bodies such as your national association of dieticians, medical and scientific research, etc. These vested interests have effectively gagged the people in power in these structures so that you get misinformed and misled and never learn the truth. It's high time you stopped listening to voices that have been blatantly compromised and start listening to your own inner voice, your gut instinct.

It's important to trust in Nature and in your own true nature, i.e. your gut feeling, and lead your life in as true and as wholesome a way as possible. Take control of your diet and move it slowly away from packaged food to food that grows in the fields. Become less reliant on supermarkets and more reliant on fresh foodstuffs. This will not only benefit your health, but that of your offspring for many generations to come, as you will read about in this book.

Food must be grown, collected, cooked and eaten in a more respectful and more spiritual way – respectful of the earth or soil it's grown in and respectful of the physical body it's put into. In contrasting the way of life in Africa and Europe, it's apparent that there is a distinct lack of spiritual wisdom guiding Western society, which is controlled by short-term gain – money. However, this is about to change. The structures are beginning to crumble and will be replaced with a simpler system. In the meantime, free yourself of any dependence you may have on these structures and feed your body **good food**.

JOHN McKENNA
THE FOOD CLINIC
E-MAIL: thefoodclinic7@gmail.com

Chapter 1
My Own Diet

GROWING UP IN IRELAND

I suppose the best place to start discussing diet and food is to examine the diet I grew up with, what I experienced in Africa and then what changes I saw on my return to Europe many years later.

During my lifetime, a revolution has taken place in the types of food people eat and how foods are prepared. It's light years away from my childhood experiences and even further away from the diet of most rural Africans.

I was born and brought up in the heart of the countryside in Northern Ireland, and when I say the 'heart' I mean I lived two miles from the nearest village and eight miles from the nearest town. We didn't have electricity for the first 11 years of my life. We used Tilley lamps and paraffin lamps as a source of light and we used an Aga stove fuelled with anthracite to heat the house and the water as well as to cook food.

My mother was a nurse and had a keen interest in nutrition. She prepared most of the food in the house and made sure that everything was as natural as possible. To give you a good idea of her obsession with good health, she used to give me a raw egg beaten in milk, much to my disgust, most mornings before I went to school. We all got a daily dose of cod liver oil and a dessertspoonful of Scott's Emulsion. She took great care to buy the best food possible and in so doing educated me about what constitutes good food.

We got most of the staples like eggs, chicken, milk, butter, vegetables and potatoes from the local farmers, so the produce was fresh but mostly organic as well. All other foods were bought once a week, usually on market day, in the local town. My mother was a very good cook and loved baking too and so made most of our bread and tarts and cakes. We therefore had a very simple but very healthy diet.

Breakfast usually consisted of a boiled egg and brown soda bread or porridge with raw milk and some honey, or occasionally sausages and bacon and black pudding with bread and butter. In those days many people made their own butter in big churns and the butter was a deep yellow colour, as the dairy cattle grazed on natural pastures. Animal produce featured heavily in the diet, as did bread and butter. We had jams and marmalade and honey to sweeten things a bit. As I grew older and had some say in what I ate, breakfast cereals such as cornflakes and All-Bran appeared. My mother was quite strict about processed food, so there wasn't a whole lot of it in our cupboards. She was also strict about the use of table sugar and preferred to use honey.

When I came home from school there was always a big pot of soup simmering on the stove. I used to have two bowls of soup with a sandwich or plain bread followed by a cooked meal. Tea was something small, like a salad, an omelette or a fry. There was seldom starch with this evening meal. My mother believed in the saying 'eat breakfast like a king, eat lunch like a prince and eat supper like a pauper', so the evening meal was light and easy to digest. We drank tea for the most part in our house.

Opposite my home there was a grocery shop where we used to buy bits and bobs. During the long summer holidays I worked in the shop serving customers, filling tea bags and sugar bags from big wooden tea chests and large paper sugar bags. The owners of the shop also had a delivery van, a mobile shop that would visit even more remote areas of the country. I loved going on this van, as it was like a big adventure. I also got to meet some interesting and some very strange people. For all the work I did I was paid not in cash, but in sweets and chocolate, usually a few bars of chocolate and a few packets of spangles, fruit gums or pastilles. On returning home I was careful to hide these away from my mother in case she took exception to the sugar overload. My maternal grandmother, who lived a mile away from us and whom we visited often, used to tell us to save all our sweets for Sunday, which was a good idea in theory but a horrible idea in practice. To me, treats were to be enjoyed immediately; I wasn't a fan of delayed gratification.

However, since I spent most of my spare time in this shop I slowly became addicted to sugar. By the time I was in my teens, I suffered from hypoglycaemic spells if I went too long without a sugar fix. I used to get a hollow feeling in my stomach and would feel a bit weak and spacey and I realised I needed to eat something quickly. My mother was worried I may have been developing diabetes, but I knew the real reason: I was eating too much sugar. I then began to take sugar in my tea, which I hadn't done when I was younger. I soon ended up taking six teaspoons per cup, until one year I decided to give up sugar for Lent (thank goodness for Lent!) and kicked the habit. Since then I've had to be very careful to avoid sugar as much as possible.

In the local town my mother would visit the greengrocer, the butcher and the bakery. It was only much later that she did some of her shopping in the supermarket. She knew the butcher very well and knew that they reared their own livestock and so trusted them to provide good-quality meat, which they always did. She bought a few cakes and some bread at the baker and lots of fruits at the greengrocer as well as a few vegetables she had problems getting from the local farmers. We didn't eat pasta or rice; it was always potatoes.

All the locals drank unpasteurised raw milk. At primary school I got bottled milk at break. Later we got deliveries of milk from the local milkman, which came in glass bottles with the cream on top. Usually the birds got to the milk first and treated themselves to a little of this cream. At that time I didn't realise just how important this cream was. It's the single most important part of the milk, but I'll explain that later in the book.

When I moved away from home to attend university, I lost my way in dietary terms and started to eat rubbish. My diet was white bread and tea for breakfast, cheese and bread for lunch and pizza or a burger for supper. Occasionally I had a proper cooked meal, but heavily laden with potatoes to fill me up. After a few months of eating like that I began to feel lethargic and mentally sluggish. It took a while to discover what was wrong, but eventually the penny dropped: there was no fresh food in my diet.

I began to eat fruits, salads and vegetables and less sugar and starch. The improvement was immediate. This was the first time I saw the beneficial effects of altering my diet. A seed had been sown.

During my long summer holidays I used to go work in New York to make some money. At the end of the summer I travelled up to Canada for a few weeks to see my sister and her husband, who lived in northern Ontario. New York was always very hot and humid during the summer so it was a great relief to get out of the city and up to the refreshing climate of Canada.

The quality of the food, in particular the bread, milk, eggs, meat and chicken, was shocking in the whole of North America. The factory-made white sliced pan was soft and spongy, like eating marshmallow. It didn't resemble the bread I had grown up with. The supermarket milk had no cream on top, as it had been homogenised. It didn't taste like milk, but more like flavoured water.

For the most part, all the delis and supermarkets had the same types of poor-quality foods. The best I could get was German rye bread in a deli close to where I stayed, so I mostly lived on sandwiches with the occasional burger or hot dog. I was also shocked at all the convenience foods available and all the fast food outlets. Virtually all the foodstuff was processed and real food was hard to find. To see people eating donuts and coffee for breakfast was new to me. Little did I know the same trends were about to follow me back to Europe.

AFRICA

After graduating from university I set off to work in West Africa on a two-year government contract. It was an exciting adventure for me, as I'd always wanted to travel and Africa was as far as my imagination stretched. Going to West Africa was a bit like going to another planet. Everything was so strange and different. It was very disorientating, as there was nothing I could identify with. Even the shades of green were different. Most importantly, the people were very different, as was the food they ate. The latter in particular took a lot of getting used to.

On arrival I was forced to eat local foods until I got settled and got my own paraffin fridge and stove. I was living in a remote area, so there was no access to Western foods. For the first two weeks I ate fufu with yams almost every night. It wasn't well accepted by my stomach, as I had severe diarrhoea for those initial few weeks. West Africans use chillies in most of their dishes and the hotter the chilli, the better. When I got my house in order I was able to cook for myself – not that I was a good cook, but at least I could control what entered my stomach. Anything was better than being at the mercy of chilli.

Breakfast usually consisted of fruits such as pawpaw (papaya), mango, pineapple or plantain fried in palm oil, which was really tasty and sweet. Lunch was usually rice and chicken or yams with meat or chicken. I didn't eat a lot of meat, as I had picked up a tapeworm after eating meat in a government rest-house (a bush motel). Plus seeing meat in the market covered in flies did nothing to enhance the image in my mind. Milk was delivered every day to my door. The beautiful Fulani women used to visit my house on their way to the local market, carrying calabashes containing milk on their heads, which was for sale in the market. It was like having the milkman (milkwoman in this case) drive past your door every day and drop off some free supplies.

The Fulani in West Africa are like the Masai of East Africa in that they are nomadic cattle herders. They are a fascinating race of people. They don't have the typical negroid features of other tribes in West Africa, but instead have more Arabic features: they have long faces and are very slender and athletic in build. From a dietary point of view they are also very different, as they live mainly on milk, meat and fruits. The Masai of East Africa live almost exclusively on milk, meat and blood as well as what grows wild in the bush, such as seeds, nuts and fruits. Both tribes are extremely healthy despite having such a restricted diet.

Once a month I made a trip to Jos, a city high up on a plateau. Not only was it a lot cooler there, but there were also supermarkets with foods imported from Europe. This was like heaven to me, as I didn't have to haggle over the price of everything and there were foods that I was used to from back home. In addition, the food was safe to eat. I would load the car with what I interpreted as 'real food' and head back to the bush. In essence, my diet was a mixture of local foods combined with Western processed foods, but it was mainly local foods.

Because of its geographical location, Nigeria has a range of both tropical and subtropical foods as well as imported foods from the Arab countries to the north. The main cereals are rice, millet, maize and sorghum. Often these cereals are used to supplement a meal such as yam with stew. Sorghum and maize can also be used to make a porridge in the same way that we use oats to make porridge. Cereals are grown locally by farmers, but in the traditional way and not using fertilisers or chemical sprays. They are grown mainly for personal use and any excess is sold in the local market. Industrialised farming methods had not arrived in West Africa when I was there in the late 1970s.

A whole host of vegetables are used as well, some of which I wasn't aware of, such as black-eyed peas, aubergine, pumpkin, squash and okra. The main root vegetables grown throughout West Africa include yams, sweet potatoes, cassava and coco-yams; these are often used as the starch component of a meal. Goat meat is very common, as is mutton, beef and chicken. In almost every cooked dish there will be peanuts as well as the trio of tomatoes, onion and chillies. Many fruits, seeds and nuts are also available. West Africans eat a lot of food, but it's all natural and grown locally using traditional methods. They have three square meals a day.

I was genuinely surprised by the range of foods available and how plentiful it was. I had had a mental image of starving Africans living in poverty. Nigeria was a wealthy country with more than enough food to feed its people. It's the fifth largest producer of oil in the world and is far from being poor. I was also impressed with the level of people's health. There was little evidence of the degenerative disorders so common in Europe, such as arthritis, hypertension, heart disease, asthma, etc. There were many infections, however, including nasty ones such as hepatitis B, a viral illness that killed two of my friends, and lots of parasites, such as malaria, bilharzia, sleeping sickness and worm infestations. West Africa is still the white man's grave, as I witnessed myself. It's quite a dangerous place to live. I lost a friend to malaria. Most of us from Europe got malaria but coped well with injections of chloroquine.

If you ignore the infections and parasites, West Africans are largely very healthy and full of life. Despite the heat they have good energy levels, love to party and can dance all night long. Life begins just before dawn – the cocks begin to crow around

5 a.m. This took a lot of getting used to, especially as it's often hard to sleep well because of the heat. Life goes on throughout the day, with a siesta for two hours in the afternoon, until late in the evening. Clearly your health has to be reasonable if you can wake before dawn, work all day, cope with the heat and still have energy to party.

I learned a lot in West Africa. In the village where I lived there were no lawyers, judges, courts, police, banks, building societies or other trappings of Western society. If there were any problems, they were sorted out by the chief. If you wanted to build a house the chief allocated you a piece of land and everyone in the village helped you build it. They don't own land as such, as the land is in the care of the chief. Nowadays the power of the local chief has been diminished as Western values have invaded these traditional societies.

I then travelled to other parts of West Africa and to Cameroon. The diet and customs were very similar through-out the region; only the language changed. Later I lived in central and then in southern Africa. Maize is the principal cereal there and there is less use of hot spices such as chilli peppers; otherwise, the diet is the same. The further south you go in Africa, the more Western the diet becomes, mainly because this is where you find the greatest concentration of white people. In Zimbabwe, Namibia and South Africa there is the same range of processed foods as found in Europe. The presence of processed foods, especially those with sugar, coincided with the presence of degenerative diseases. In southern Africa, if black people abandoned their traditional diet in favour of processed foods such as refined maize meal, white flour and sugar, they inevitably started to manifest diabetes, hypertension, heart disease, allergies and so on. This pattern was most noticeable in the black townships around major urban centres such as Harare, Johannesburg and Cape Town, where blacks presented with diseases previously found only in the white population.

RETURN TO EUROPE

After many years in different parts of Africa, I returned to Europe in 2002. I moved to England, as my daughter was living there at the time. I was shocked by what I saw. The average person in the street of the local town where I was living was visibly overweight, many of the children at the local school were overweight and even the babies were on the plump side. Clearly, something very unusual had been going on in the 1980s and 90s while I was in Africa.

On my visit to the supermarket, I began to see what was wrong. The foods that filled people's shopping trolleys were mainly processed foods and mostly carbohydrates – pizza, waffles, breads, biscuits, cakes, pancakes, breakfast cereals, snack foods, etc. – and all laden with sugar. Even worse, people were eating either convenience foods such as pies, burgers, chips and takeaways or ready-made meals or microwave dinners. There was little or no fresh food in the diet. The diet I grew up on and the traditional diet I experienced in different parts of Africa were now replaced with factory foods. These were foods that were not designed by Nature, but by food chemists. These foods were destroying whole populations.

I couldn't believe what I was witnessing. To this day I'm still in a state of shock at how radically our diet has been transformed in such a short space of time.

With a little bit of research it became clear that the obesity crisis began in the mid-1970s in the US and in the early 1980s in Europe. This coincided with the removal of fat from foods in the mid-1970s and the addition of high fructose corn syrup to replace the fat. It was known in the 1950s and 60s that fructose causes obesity and I had learned this at college in Dublin in the early 1970s. It must have also been known to the food chemists who decided to replace fat with fructose. Why allow such an international catastrophe like this to happen? Making money for food companies is clearly more important than people's health.

What still astonishes me is the impotence of politicians, doctors, dieticians and international organisations such as the World Health Organization (WHO) to deal with the obesity epidemic. Unfortunately, they have become part of the problem. Most organisations dealing with the epidemic are sponsored by the same food companies that are causing the problem. When the WHO decided to inform people to cut sugar out of their diet, they were promptly told by a member of the US government to change their minds or their budget would be cut, so the WHO altered their advice. Needless to say, the public wasn't informed and everyone became aware of the power of the food companies over politicians.

Everywhere in the world where Western processed foods are sold, there is an obesity epidemic. It has nothing to do with lack of exercise or with fat in the diet and everything to do with sugary foodstuffs. To advise people to avoid fat, eat more carbohydrate and exercise is tantamount to deliberately making people ill. What is the motivation for such advice? All it does is discredit the whole of the establishment. It discredits politicians, government advisors, food manufacturers, dieticians and doctors as well as medical and scientific research.

The purpose of this book is to try to bring some common sense back and to help people reverse the trends of the 1980s and 90s. It's designed to get you back to a more natural diet and to reduce your dependence on supermarkets. It's written to help you distinguish between real food and food devoid of nutrition.

Chapter 2
Two Amazing Researchers

INTRODUCTION

'Man is the only species clever enough to make his own food and stupid enough to eat it.'
— BARRY GROVES

A wiser quote I have never read. Man has become separate from and detached from Nature, and all within a short space of time. It began after the Second World War but has accelerated during my lifetime, i.e. over the last 60 years. From my childhood, when I got fresh produce from a local farm, I'm now reduced to being dependent on supermarkets to feed myself. This has occurred in the last 40 years in particular, as the supermarket chains began to put the smaller shops out of business. It was a gradual, insidious process. Local greengrocers, butchers, bakers, etc. were replaced with impersonal self-help chains of superstores, which were, and still are, more interested in profit than in providing good food. Never mind the quality, look at the price. To quote from the movie *Food, Inc.,* 'bigger, fatter, cheaper, faster' is the motto for chickens given animal feed containing antibiotics and growth hormone and reared in inhumane conditions. These kinds of chickens are preferred to free-range, humanely raised chickens, as there is more profit in the former.

The big retailers such as Tesco in the UK and Ireland have gradually gained power over the farmers and dictate what to do and how to do it.

Government and European Union regulations have also done their bit in this chain of events by standardising the size, shape and colour of our foods. This has led to a rapid decline in the quality of our food. It's time for us all to come to our senses and reverse things while it's still possible. Spend a little time and energy finding a farmer who will sell you produce directly from his or her farm. Alternatively, get a plot of ground or an allotment and teach yourself and your children to grow food. Learn how to make yoghurt, butter and bread as your mother or grandmother may have done. If you can't do any of this, at least stop shopping in the supermarket or wean yourself off supermarket dependence and support your local butcher, baker or local market instead. Do something, and most importantly, explain to your children why you're doing it so that they will adopt good shopping habits when they're adults.

The importance of doing this will become evident to you by the end of this chapter. I have dedicated this chapter to the work of two brilliant men who researched nutrition over 70 years ago. They were both American and were both aware of the negative impact of processed foods on the health of both humans and animals. They carried out some incredible research in the 1930s, the results of which are as relevant (if not more so) today as they were back then. This research is worth learning about and keeping at the forefront of your mind every time you go hunting for food in your local shops.

DR WESTON A. PRICE

I'll begin with the work of Dr Weston A. Price, as the results will leave you in no doubt about the role processed food is playing in our modern health problems.

Dr Price wasn't a doctor or a dietician or a nutritionist, but rather, a dentist. However, he had a wonderful knowledge of nutrition, and after his travels around the world studying various population groups he gained quite a reputation for his success at treating medical conditions with nutritional advice. Dr Price practised as a dentist in Cleveland, Ohio, and saw first hand the deterioration in the dental health of his patients with the advent of modern foods in the early 1900s. Dr Price decided to visit and study the healthiest people on the planet in order to study their diet in detail and then use this knowledge to help his own patients. Little did he know that the tide of deterioration he was witnessing in the 1920s was to continue for another 90 years, culminating in an obesity epidemic.

He began his travels in 1931 and continued to travel over the next 10 years, by which point he had accumulated more data than any other researcher of his time. He had documented detail not just on the incidence of dental caries (tooth decay), dental arches and facial structure, but on the general health and especially the nutrition of each group of people he visited. What amazed me on reading his book *Nutrition and Physical Degeneration* was how simple their diet was and how few foods they ate. This shouldn't have been such a revelation to me, as I had spent enough time with primitive tribes in Africa to realise that this was the case. For example, some of the people he visited ate only oats and fish for the most part and were perfectly healthy – that is, there was little fruit and vegetables in the diet (no five a day for them, I'm afraid).

Dr Price was asking the basic question as to why there was so much dental decay, crowding of teeth, high dental arches and increased susceptibility to infection, especially tuberculosis, which was prevalent at the time. His nephew worked for *National Geographic* and was very helpful in finding isolated peoples with perfect teeth and excellent health and where there was no doctor or dentist.

He began in 1931 by travelling to an isolated community in the Loetschental Valley high up in the Alps in Switzerland. This community was so isolated that they had to depend solely on local foods, so they had no exposure to modern processed foods. He studied all 2,000 inhabitants of the valley. They had excellent overall health, no cases of tuberculosis, almost zero incidence of dental caries (0.3 per cent) and ate a very simple diet of sourdough rye bread, cheese and raw goat milk or cow milk and meat once a week – a diet rich in saturated fat, for those of you who still believe saturated fat is bad for you. The men in this valley were known throughout Europe for their great physical strength and were chosen to be trained as the well-known Swiss Guards who protect the Pope in the Vatican. Dr Price examined the teeth of every child in the valley and made careful notes to record his findings. His wife helped with the collection and filing of data. He also listed and took samples of the foods they ate and sent these samples to his laboratory in Cleveland for analysis.

What is most interesting about their diet are the following details:

- They had little or no fruit and vegetables.
- They ate lots of animal (saturated) fat.
- They pre-digested the rye before eating it.
- They wouldn't eat lean meat without the fat and they consumed all the organs, including the adrenals, kidneys, heart, eyes, brain and the lining of the gut. These were the most treasured parts of the animal.
- The milk was raw (i.e. unpasteurised).

The pastures on which the goats and cattle grazed were quite special. According to Dr Price's findings, the grass was rich in chlorophyll (the green pigment in green plants), making it particularly nutritious. Substances rich in chlorophyll, such as spirulina and *Chlorella*, are highly rated in the world of nutrition, as they're so full of vitamins and minerals. In winter they fed the animals dried grass (hay) and in spring took the cattle high up to eat the fresh grass fed by melting ice.

These people were effectively cut off from contact with other villages, as they were surrounded on three sides by very high mountains and on the fourth side by a track that was impassable for most of the year, and then only on foot. No vehicles could access the village, so there were no modern foods such as white bread, sugar, biscuits, cakes, tinned foods and soft drinks. How fortunate these people were, and how healthy. Dr Price had truly found an isolated village. He was amazed at the exceptional level of good health among the population as well as good dental health despite there not being a toothbrush in sight. He photographed many of them, and on examining the photos it's apparent that they had perfectly formed teeth: no crowding of the teeth, normal, low dental arches (what we non-dentists would call the palate or roof of the mouth) and broad facial bones that allowed room for all the teeth, including the wisdom teeth. They didn't brush their teeth at all and so the teeth had a covering or residue, but no evidence of infection or plaque. Their immunity to all infections, including tuberculosis, which was killing people down in the lowlands of Switzerland and indeed in the rest of Europe, was remarkable. Dr Price attributed their wonderful health to their simple, natural diet.

He then moved to another mountain village, Vissoie, which was quite similar to the previous village except that a road connected the village to the rest of the country and so they had access to a modern bakery (white bread, biscuits, cakes), sweetened jams, jellies, etc. In Vissoie the incidence of dental caries was 2.3 per cent, which means that 23 people per thousand of the population had evidence of previous or present tooth decay, compared with only three per thousand in the Loetschental Valley. The diet of the people in Vissoie was very similar to that in the previous village except that they had access to refined carbohydrates. The introduction of modern processed foods lowered their immunity not only to dental decay, but to other infections as well, notably tuberculosis. It also led to the development of chronic degenerative diseases such as arthritis and heart disease.

He then moved to the world-famous health resort of St Moritz, where the diet was almost totally modern. There, the rate of dental caries was 29 per cent, or 290 per thousand of the population, and tuberculosis was rampant. The only children with good teeth in St Moritz were those who had moved down from the remote mountain villages and had retained a natural diet.

In the area around Lake Constance in the lowlands of Switzerland, Dr Price recorded a very high rate of dental caries – almost 100 per cent. In the TB clinics in this area, none of the patients were from the high mountain valleys, suggesting that these mountain people had a much greater resistance to infection. However, this resistance began to disappear upon the introduction of modern processed foods, and when the natural parts of the diet were eventually replaced completely by modern foods, the body began to manifest what we now regard as commonplace disorders: infections, blocked arteries, osteoarthritis and asthma. He was beginning to prove to himself and others just how critical a role diet plays in human health. He was now excited to test these findings in other isolated locations in the world.

Next on his list of places to visit were the islands of the Outer Hebrides, where the people were also famed for their good health, fine teeth, strong physiques and cheerful dispositions. This was of particular interest to me, as I'm Irish and have always been impressed with the high level of health of people from the isolated parts of Ireland, especially the islands such as Achill Island just off the Atlantic coast.

Dr Price travelled to the Isle of Lewis, which had a population of 20,000, who were mostly involved in fishing or were sheepherders. They lived in small thatched cottages. Not much grew on the island, as there was little lime (calcium) and therefore the soil was fairly infertile. As a consequence, there were few trees, no fruits and little in the way of vegetables. Most of the island was peat bog. Because of the poor quality of the soil, very few cattle could be raised (only some on a government experimental farm); hence, there was little or no dairy produce either. Oat was the only crop that would grow, so the bulk of the diet was seafood and oats; very occasionally there was a little barley. Oats were used to make porridge and oat cakes, which were eaten with most meals. Lots of fish, lobsters, oysters, crabs and clams were also consumed. The liver of the codfish was a prized food and was fed to pregnant women and growing children. (Now you know why my mother used to give me cod liver oil.) The fishermen and women often worked from 6 a.m. to 10 p.m., as there were large quantities of fish to be prepared and packed for shipping to the mainland; they had amazing energy reserves. The thatched roof of the cottages was replaced every October and the old thatch was used as fertiliser for the soil, as the locals knew it contained something that helped the oats to grow.

Like in Switzerland, the more isolated the people, the lower the rate of dental decay. In Stornoway, the capital, many young people had false teeth due to the high incidence of tooth decay. TB was common in Stornoway but virtually absent among the isolated people. The negative effects of modern foods were all too apparent. Dr Price also visited the Isle of Harris and noted the exact same patterns: the more isolated the people, the better their level of health.

This is quite remarkable when you think of how limited the diet of these people was – they were eating little more than seafood and oats. This flies in the face of everything we've been taught about the importance of dairy and the so-called five a day of fruit and vegetables. Clearly, the body functions in a different way. The body seems to respond best to natural foods and seems to malfunction as soon as processed foods are introduced. The exact details of the diet are almost less important, in that the isolated Swiss people were eating rye bread and dairy, while the Celts were eating seafood and oats. If I were to put you on either of these diets I would be accused of causing malnutrition. Yet how come these people not only had no deficiency diseases, but were actually thriving? Now you see why I find the work of this man so fascinating. He revealed many uncomfortable truths about the role of diet in human health, and more importantly, human ill health.

Next, Dr Price visited the Eskimo population of Alaska. He described the Eskimo as the last of the Stone Age people, through whom we have access to a truly ancestral way of life. They are the last of the races of people who thrived in the harsh Arctic environment, where temperatures can dip to a staggering −70 degrees Celsius. It's impossible to grow anything in an environment as hostile as this, so their diet didn't include cereals, vegetables or fruits and also excluded dairy, as there is no livestock at such latitudes. Again, despite such a restricted diet they exhibited excellent physical health, amazing physical strength, dental perfection and a complete absence of tuberculosis. Dr Price reported that a typical Eskimo man can carry 100 pounds of weight for a considerable distance in both arms and between his teeth.

Upon contact with the white man and his food, which was referred to as 'store grub', the Eskimos' health deteriorated. The typical diet of the Eskimo consisted of salmon, seal oil, which is rich in vitamin A, occasional caribou, kelp, groundnuts and occasional berries. All organs of the fish and caribou were eaten. The most prized food was salmon eggs, again reserved for pregnant women and young children. The bulk of their diet was fish protein, fish oils and seal oil.

A very isolated group of Eskimos was studied at Stoney River and were found to have an incidence of dental caries of 0.3 per cent, while a group on Nelson Island in the Bering Sea had an incidence of 0.1 per cent. Children at a Catholic school in Holy Cross, Alaska, where all bar one had access to modern foods, had an incidence of 18.7 per cent, confirming the key role of diet in the health of these people. Again, exposure to modern foods led to changes in the facial bone structure of children and as a consequence changes in the shape of the dental arch. This was often combined with increased susceptibility to infection and to degenerative disorders.

One of the most beloved men in Alaska at that time was Dr Joseph Romig, who worked as a doctor in the hospital in Anchorage. He had 36 years' experience working closely with the Eskimo and Native American populations. He witnessed a high incidence of gall bladder problems, stomach and intestinal issues and the need for appendix operations in those on a modern diet, yet none of these problems were an issue with the races on a traditional diet.

He also saw a high incidence of malignant disease (that is, cancer) in those eating refined foods and a zero incidence of malignancy among those eating a purely natural diet. He treated tuberculosis via diet: he put his patients on the diet discussed above or sent them back to an isolated village if they had relatives there. He solved many medical issues simply by altering his patients' diet. He was a great believer in natural methods of healing. Because of his success in treating tuberculosis in this way, he became very well known and respected.

In 1933 Dr Price moved to northern British Columbia and the Yukon Territory to study the Native Americans who lived there. They lived away from the coastal areas and thus didn't have access to seafood. As temperatures were very low there, like in Alaska, it wasn't possible to grow foods such as vegetables, fruits or cereals or to keep livestock such as cattle, goats or sheep.

These people existed mostly on wild game such as moose, caribou and bears, yet they didn't suffer from deficiencies in their diet. When Dr Price asked how they avoided scurvy, they described how they used various parts of the animal, such as the adrenals and the wall of the second stomach of the moose, for vitamin C. They seemed to have a wealth of knowledge and an understanding of Nature's secrets. They were skilled at building wooden cabins to withstand the bitter cold of these latitudes and had herbal cures for a wide range of problems. When Dr Price asked why they didn't share their knowledge and wisdom with the white man, the chief replied that the white man knew too much to ask the Indian anything. Western culture is indeed very arrogant and looks down on the very people who lived in harmony with Nature for so long on this planet, but soon, as Western culture collapses and the money games come to an end, we will have to revert to a simpler and more natural way of being and so will need the wisdom and knowledge of these people.

Like all the other isolated peoples who survived on a purely natural diet, the Indians of northern Canada had an almost zero rate of dental caries. They also had no evidence of tuberculosis, osteoarthritis or any other degenerative diseases. Later, Dr Price was able to visit Indians in other parts of Canada who lived on reservations; he quotes his findings from the biggest reservation in Canada, which is in Brantford, Ontario.

Alcoholism was widespread, as were degenerative disorders and a significant number of maternity issues. Dental caries was rampant. These settled Indians had all the privileges of modern life, including a modern hospital, but no amount of modernity could halt the steady deterioration in their health. Dr Price attributed this deterioration to the readily available supply of modern foods, especially refined carbohydrates such as white bread, cakes, biscuits, soft drinks and sweetened foods. His study included documenting the rate of caries in a training school on the reservation, but what's interesting about this school is that the students were fed raw milk, wholewheat bread, lots of fresh fruit and vegetables and no refined carbohydrates. They had very few medical or dental problems, which confirms the fact that diet is the single most important contributing factor to good health. This is further borne out when skulls are compared in Vancouver Museum, where there is no evidence of dental caries in the skulls of primitive people compared to a rate of 38 per cent among the skulls of modern natives. Modern foods wreak havoc in the bodies of all who consume them.

Dr Price visited many other parts of the world, including Polynesia, Melanesia, Australian Aboriginals, different parts of Africa, New Zealand and Peru. In total he visited 14 different isolated locations. The same patterns were observed in each place: in places where the native diet was replaced with modern foods, the rate of dental caries, tuberculosis and degenerative diseases rose sharply.

The tests performed on primitive foods in his laboratory looked at the levels of various micronutrients (vitamins and minerals). He also looked at the levels of vitamins and minerals in plant-based foods compared to animal-based foods and had some very interesting things to say. He paid a lot of attention to what he called the fat-soluble activators, i.e. the fat-soluble vitamins, as these formed a key component of the primitive people's diet. He found that without an adequate supply of these vitamins it isn't possible to absorb sufficient levels of calcium and phosphorus, which are critical for growth. In other words, children may be eating foods with calcium, but because of a lack of vitamins, they may actually be starved of calcium because they're unable to absorb it. For example, vitamin D assists the absorption of calcium in the gut.

He compared the Eskimo diet to a modern diet and found that the Eskimo diet had 10 times more fat-soluble vitamins, 5.4 times as much calcium, 7.9 times as much magnesium and 49 times as much iodine. The Eskimo diet was far superior to the modern diet in every respect. His comparison of the diet of all the other primitive peoples proved the same thing. Dr Price was suggesting that the effects of a deficient diet have far-reaching effects not just on one's physical health, but on one's mental, emotional and spiritual well-being. I couldn't agree with him more. The Native American Indians alluded to the damaging effects of sugar in the white man's diet, saying it weakens the mind and the spirit.

Dr Price has some interesting stories to tell and I'd like to share a few with you now, as they will confirm your belief in the role of simple nutrition. A young boy who was suffering severe convulsions was brought to Dr Price's office. The church minister who brought him felt that the problem was nutritional and thought Dr Price could help. The boy's convulsions had been getting progressively worse over the previous eight months. His diet consisted of white bread and skimmed milk, as the family was poor. Dr Price felt that his convulsions were due to a low calcium level in his blood. Dr Price changed his diet to wheat gruel made from freshly ground wheat and whole milk containing the fat, as well as the addition of a high-vitamin butter with each meal. When given this food for the first time, he slept all night without a convulsion. He was fed the same food five times the next day, and still no convulsion. He recovered quite quickly and regained full health. By giving the child simple, natural food, the body made a remarkable recovery.

This story is relevant to modern times, as many children are given skimmed milk or low-fat milk. It's true that the calcium that the boy needed was in the watery skimmed milk. However, to absorb it you also need vitamin D, which is in the fat portion of the milk – vitamin D is fat soluble and so is found in animal fats. This is why saturated or animal fat is so critical for human health. Humans can't make vitamin D, so we have to obtain it from food. Guinea pigs, however, make their own vitamin D, which is why they are used as a source of food in Peru, especially high up in the Andes, where there is no dairy produce available.

The next story is quoted directly from Dr Price's book (2008) (reprinted with permission from the Price-Pottenger Nutrition Foundation):

Shortly before our arrival in Northern Canada a white prospector had died of scurvy. Beside him was his white man's packet of canned foods. Any Indian man or woman, boy or girl could have told him how to save his life by eating animal organs or the buds of trees.

Another illustration of the wisdom of the native Indians of that far north country came to me through two prospectors whom we rescued and brought out with us just before the fall freeze-up. They had gone into the district which at that time was still unchartered and unsurveyed, to prospect for precious metals and radium. They were both doctors of engineering and science and had been sent with very elaborate equipment from one of the large national mining corporations. Owing to the inaccessibility of the region, they adopted a plan for reaching it quickly. They had flown across the two ranges of mountains from Alaska and when they arrived at the inside range i.e. the Rocky Mountain range, they found the altitude so high that their plane could not fly over the range and, as a result, they were brought down on a little lake outside. The plane then returned but was unable to reach the outside world because of shortage of fuel. The pilot had to leave it on a waterway and trudge over the mountains to civilisation. The two prospectors undertook to carry their equipment and provisions over the Rocky Mountain range into the interior district where they were to prospect. They found the distance across the plateau to be about one hundred miles and the elevation ranging up to nine thousand feet. While they had provisions and equipment to stay two years they found it would take all of this time to carry all of their provisions and instruments across this plateau. They accordingly abandoned everything and rather than remain in the country with very uncertain facilities and prospects for obtaining food and shelter, made a forced march to the Liard River with the hope that some expedition might be in that territory. One of the men told me the following tragic story. While they were crossing the high plateau he nearly went blind with so violent a pain in his eyes that he feared he would go insane. It was not snow blindness, for they were equipped with glasses. It was xerophthalmia, due to lack of vitamin A. One day he almost ran into a mother grizzly bear and her two cubs. Fortunately, they did not attack him but moved off. He sat down on a stone and wept in despair of ever seeing his family again. As he sat there holding his throbbing head, he heard a voice and looked up. It was an old Indian who had been tracking that grizzly bear. He recognised this prospector's plight and while neither could understand the language of the other, the Indian after making an examination of his eyes, took him by the hand and led him to a stream that was coursing its way down the mountain. Here as the prospector sat waiting the Indian built a trap of stones across the stream. He then went upstream and waded down splashing as he came and thus drove the trout into the trap. He threw the fish out on the bank and told the prospector to eat the flesh of the head and the tissues at the back of the eyes with the result that in a few hours his pain had largely subsided. In one day his sight was rapidly returning and in two days his eyes were nearly normal. He told me with profound emotion and gratitude that that Indian had certainly saved his life.

Now modern science knows that one of the richest sources of vitamin A in the entire animal body is that of the tissues at the back of the eyes, including the retina.

This book is a treasure trove of information that is infinitely more valuable today, since we are in the midst of self-destruction in the form of an obesity epidemic. The information in this book is helpful in guiding us all back to a simple, natural diet and a simple, natural way of life.

DR FRANCIS M. POTTENGER

The other bit of research I'd like to discuss is the work of Dr Francis M. Pottenger. He worked as a doctor in a sanatorium in Monrovia, California, treating tuberculosis, asthma and other respiratory disorders. He worked in this sanatorium during the 1930s, at the same time as Dr Price's travels. In fact, the two knew each other as both had a keen interest in nutrition, especially the role of the modern diet in the onset of degenerative diseases.

Dr Pottenger used to treat his patients with raw foods and adrenal gland extract. He was so impressed with the benefits of this treatment that he decided to do nutritional experiments on donated cats. These experiments took place over a 10-year period between 1931 and 1941 and involved 900 cats in all.

His first bit of research looked at the effects of cooked meat versus raw meat on the cats' health. One group of cats was given a diet of two-thirds raw meat, one-third raw milk and a little cod liver oil, while the second group was given the same diet except that the meat was cooked. The cats in the first group were very healthy, as were their kittens of each successive generation. The cats in the second group, who were fed cooked meat, didn't do as well and had a variety of health problems, mainly degenerative diseases later in life. The third generation also had health problems, such as weakness, poor co-ordination and degenerative diseases earlier in life. The fourth generation died early in life and some were born with defects such as blindness. There was no fifth generation. Dr

Pottenger postulated that there must be something in raw food that was essential for the health of the cats that was being destroyed by cooking the meat. We now know that this essential ingredient is an amino acid called taurine.

He then did an experiment to test the effects of different types of milk on the cats' health. He divided the cats into three groups. The cats in group one were given two-thirds raw milk plus one-third raw meat, the cats in group two were given the same diet but the milk was pasteurised, while the type of milk used in the third group was condensed milk.

The cats in the first group had excellent health. The cats in the second group showed signs of degenerative disease and the third group had significant health problems. So the healthiest milk was raw, unpasteurised milk. This experimental evidence is used by many to promote the benefits of raw milk. It certainly ties in well with what Dr Price discovered in Switzerland and elsewhere on his travels.

Personally, I find Dr Price's research of much greater interest and of direct benefit to human health, as it's often hard to make statements on human health based on experiments on animals. Dr Price's work is of particular interest to me as I have direct experience of having lived with primitive people, who have always fascinated me. It's also of special interest because like Dr Price, I have a great interest in the effects of diet on human health. From such studies, we begin to get an appreciation of which foods to avoid and which to consume. In Chapter 4 I examine the modern diet and compare it to a healthy diet, but first, in Chapter 3 I'd like to briefly talk about something everyone is now taught: the food pyramid.

Chapter 3
The Food Pyramid

A HISTORY OF THE FOOD PYRAMID

Back in the early 1990s, the food pyramid was born in the US. Sweden produced the first ever food pyramid in the mid-1970s, but the US version has had the greatest influence on the eating habits of people in other countries.

The development of the US food pyramid had a long incubation period. Since the late 1940s, scientists and doctors wanted to know why heart disease was so prevalent in the West. By heart disease, I'm referring to coronary artery disease, which is commonly called blocked arteries. Many people were dying of heart attacks and it was the number one priority of the medical profession to find out why. Professor Ancel Keys of the University of Minnesota in the US was convinced that his research held the answer. His famous study, which got a write-up in *Time* magazine, was called the Seven Countries Study (Keys, 1970). He tried to find an association between certain factors in the participants' diet and their lifestyle to see if he could find any associations with the incidence of heart disease in the same participants. He found a clear-cut relationship between animal fat (also called saturated fat) intake and the incidence of heart attacks. He published his results and by 1952 suggested that the whole country reduce its intake of animal fat, i.e. cut down on milk, cheese, yoghurt, cream, meat, bacon, sausage, eggs, etc. Because this data tied in with information obtained from post-mortems on people who had died of a heart attack which showed a build-up of cholesterol in the walls of the coronary arteries and because it also tied in with experimental data on laboratory animals, the hypothesis that animal fat was the culprit was universally accepted until further proof emerged.

Everyone jumped on the bandwagon. Eventually the media got hold of this information and the world at large began to accept this hypothesis. Everyone began to demonise fats, especially animal fats. Then in 1961 the famous Framingham Heart Study linked elevated blood cholesterol with heart disease. Again, everyone jumped to the conclusion that animal fat intake was raising the level of cholesterol in the blood-stream and causing blockages in the arteries. Without testing this hypothesis, the American Heart Association then began actively promoting a low-fat diet. They were severely criticised for doing so, as was the government. In 1968 the government asked Senator George McGovern to chair a Select Committee on Nutrition and Human Health and produce a report. Nine years later, a report was produced that endorsed the recommendations of a low-fat diet. In one fell swoop, hypothesis had become fact.

However, in the intervening nine years a lot of research showed no link between animal fat and coronary artery disease, so Senator McGovern's report wasn't met with enthusiasm by all. In fact, there was a public outcry by many in the research community and in the farming industry. Their objections were ignored for the most part. The horse had bolted and the world gladly accepted animal fat as the demon. Essentially, from then on all food policy accepted the low-fat hypothesis as fact. Food manufacturers began to reduce the fat content of their foods, governments issued advice in the form of food pyramids and the media and advertisers did their bit. After all, what's good enough for the Americans is good enough for the rest of us, isn't it? America was a superpower in the world, there was scientific evidence to back it up and there was the report of nine years from a senator. The train was steaming down the track and we were all aboard. All advice and research and protests from objecting scientists were ignored. There was no room for party poopers on board.

Following on from this 'ploughing ahead regardless' policy, the US Department of Agriculture (USDA) decided to draw up a set of guidelines advising people what to eat and how much to eat. This has become the famous, or some would say infamous, food pyramid. There was no going back now. All the evidence was now encapsulated in one easy-to-understand diagram. Here it is in all its glory.

Have you seen this before? It's now in every hospital, doctor's surgery, nurse's room and dietician's office. It's in schoolbooks and university textbooks. It's even on some break-fast cereal boxes. Do you understand the messages it's trying to convey? Try explaining it to your partner, child or friend and see how well you understand it. For example, do you know what a serving of dairy is? That should test your knowledge.

Figure 3.1: USDA food pyramid, 1992

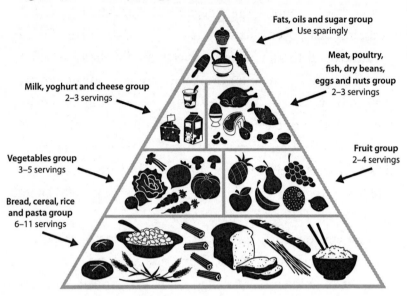

This food pyramid has become the basis for most other food pyramids in other countries. The food pyramid in your country may have slight variations, but it will essentially be the same. For example, messages such as 'five a day', meaning eat five portions of fruit and vegetables a day, are taken from the food pyramid in the UK and are now engrained in the subconscious mind of UK citizens.

Let me now try to explain the main ideas that the USDA is trying to get across. Let's start at the bottom of the pyramid.

Figure 3.2: Bread, cereal, rice and pasta group

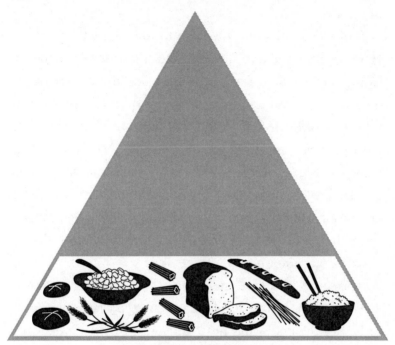

Bread, cereal, rice and pasta group
6–11 servings

As you can see from Figure 3.1, the pyramid is divided into sections, with each section representing a food group. Alongside each section is written the recommended daily intake for that food group.

The base of the pyramid, as seen in Figure 3.2, is composed of grain (breads, cereals, rice, pasta) and potatoes. These foods are also called complex carbohydrates or starchy foods. These are energy-giving foods. One serving of this food group is equivalent to a slice of bread, half a cup of cereal, one potato or three dessertspoons of rice or pasta. The pyramid suggests 6–11 servings a day. In fact, the more carbohydrates you eat, the better, which is why it's at the base of the pyramid. It suggests that carbohydrate is the single most important part of our diet.

Now let's switch our attention to the top of the pyramid. Here we find fats and oils. The fact that they're at the top would suggest that they're the least important part of our diet. The pyramid tells us to use them sparingly, meaning as little as possible. After all, fats will kill you. They will slowly create a greasy sludge, clog your arteries and strike you down when you least expect it. Notice there's no distinction between animal fats (saturated fats) and other fats. It just says use fats and oils sparingly. Sugar is also included in this food group, so you're being advised to use it sparingly as well, but it doesn't specify exact amounts.

In essence, the core message that the USDA is trying to convey is 'eat more carbohydrates and less fat if you want to be healthy and avoid heart disease'. Now let's look at the middle section of the pyramid.

Fruits and vegetables are next in order of importance, as you can see in Figure 3.3. By implication, fruits and vegetables are more important than protein and dairy, as the latter both contain animal fat. So your diet should be based on:

- Lots of grains
- Some fruit and vegetables
- Less dairy and protein
- Little or no fats, oils or sugar.

Figure 3.3: Fruit and vegetable group

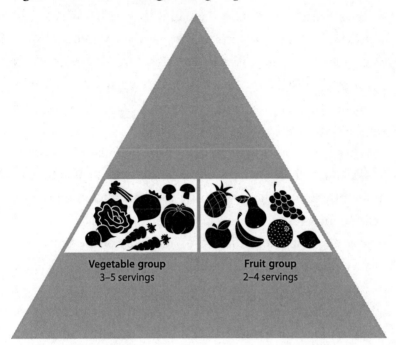

This food pyramid is promoting the idea of a low-fat diet, pure and simple. It's also blatantly promoting the food processing industry. It implies that my mother and grandmother were wrong, and for that matter your mother and grandmother too. In fact, it suggests that all cultures that have ever existed on this planet have been wrong and that many of them therefore must have suffered from clogged arteries and died of heart disease.

Seeing as how there isn't a shred of evidence to support this, there must be something fundamentally wrong with the idea that animal fat causes heart disease. Many cultures eat vast amounts of animal fat and yet have no heart disease. Heart disease only appears when these cultures adopt a

Western diet. Once these peoples start eating processed foods such as breads, biscuits, cakes, refined cereals, sweets and soft drinks, all the Western diseases – obesity, hypertension, osteoarthritis, heart disease, diabetes, etc. – appear. Look again at the list of processed foods I've just listed. They're all carbohydrates, albeit some of them have sugar, which is a simple carbohydrate.

When I first went to Africa and met the Fulani in Nigeria, I was shocked that they were so healthy and yet ate very differently to me. They ate mostly dairy produce and protein, little or no starch, no vegetables but occasional fruits and berries and nuts. According to my thinking at the time, they had a deficient diet and should have suffered from deficiency diseases. They were deprived and were waiting for the wisdom (and of course the foods) of the white man to rescue them. Little did I realise that the shoe was on the other foot. Arrogance can blind you from the truth. As soon as the Fulani or any other rural Africans moved to the city and started to consume the white man's foods, they began to suffer. I saw the exact same pattern in Zimbabwe, Botswana, Lesotho and South Africa. Having read Dr Price's book *Nutrition and Degenerative Disorders*, it's clear that modern processed foods are the root cause of most degenerative diseases and are the root cause of the obesity epidemic. To imply that animal fat, which has been a key constituent of the diet of millions of people for centuries, is in some way harming us is shifting the attention away from the real culprit, i.e. carbohydrates, and teaches people not to trust their loved ones (mothers, in this case) or their culture and not to trust in Nature. In my opinion, food manufacturers are pulling the wool over everyone's eyes and are the real driving force behind the USDA food pyramid.

To dispel any niggling thoughts that animal fat may be a problem, let's examine the evidence for and against the hypothesis that animal fat can cause heart disease.

EVIDENCE FOR: ZERO

You may be shocked to learn that there isn't a shred of hard scientific evidence linking dietary animal (saturated) fat with heart disease. However, there *is* evidence linking raised bad cholesterol (low-density lipoprotein (LDL) cholesterol) in the blood with heart disease. It isn't dietary animal fat that causes the rise in LDL cholesterol – it's sugar. This statement doesn't sit well with the food manufacturers, so it's not spoken about. It's politely swept under the carpet.

It took 11 years for the US Surgeon General's office to conclude in 1999 that there was 'insufficient' (better phrased as 'zero') evidence linking heart disease and dietary fat. Effectively, the US National Institutes of Health, the US Surgeon General's office, the American Heart Association, the US government and the medical profession have conned everyone into believing that dietary fats are a problem. An entire low-fat industry has sprung up in support of this idea. Now nobody has the courage to admit the truth, so we live and base our food intake on a lie. Lies of this magnitude discredit everyone. It's now 2013 and health officials worldwide are still promoting low-fat diets. I guess the runaway train is too far down the track to stop it.

In summary, the food pyramids are wrong, as there is no medical or scientific evidence to support them. However, this doesn't stop government bodies from producing new ones. In

2012 the USDA decided to add insult to injury by producing a food plate instead of a pyramid. This food plate is as ridiculous as the original food pyramid. Stop with the food plates and pyramids! People aren't stupid. We have survived without the advice of organisations such as the USDA for centuries. Now that we're clear that they have been dishing up (no pun intended) the wrong advice, may they swallow some humble pie (no pun intended) and choke on their own words (pun intended).

Professor Ancel Keys, who originally suggested a link between dietary fat and heart disease, has since admitted there is no link. The famous Framingham Heart Study, which has been looking at risk factors for heart disease for over 50 years, has admitted the same thing.

EVIDENCE AGAINST

I'll mention just five pieces of evidence against the link between dietary fat and heart disease, which should be enough to convince you.

1. There's no evidence of heart disease among certain populations that have a high saturated fat intake, such as the Eskimos. In Europe the French have the highest level of saturated fat in their diet, yet they have the lowest incidence of heart disease.
2. We've been advised to eat a low-fat diet for more than 30 years, but the incidence of heart disease hasn't altered significantly.
3. Rationing during the 1940s and 50s led to much less saturated fat in the diet of people in the UK. During this

period, the incidence of heart disease trebled. In other words, more than 50 million people were eating little animal fat for about 12 years, yet heart disease increased. The US government clearly didn't know this when they designed the food pyramid; nor did other governments.

4. Professor Michael Oliver, past president of the Royal College of Physicians in the UK, has openly criticised those who proposed any link between dietary fat and heart disease. He suggested there was no hard evidence linking the two.

5. Dr George Mann studied the Masai of East Africa in the 1970s. They had the highest saturated fat and cholesterol intake of any population group ever studied, yet they had no evidence of heart disease. These results were published in the *American Journal of Epidemiology* in 1972 (Mann et al., 1972). He suggested that the diet–heart hypothesis was 'the greatest scam in the history of medicine'.

Are you convinced yet? There's an overwhelming amount of evidence against the idea that dietary fat causes heart disease – so much, in fact, that one would be very reluctant to publicly suggest such a link. Yet this doesn't deter government agencies from persisting in this scam. It really is the greatest scandal and many heads need to roll.

Let's get back to the food pyramid. You may have noticed the fly in the ink by now. Do you not find it a wee bit peculiar that the first food pyramid was produced not by the WHO, the Department of Health, the Surgeon General's office or a university, but by the Department of Agriculture, whose job is to promote the food industry? I would call this a clear conflict of interest. It's a bit like me advising you to drink more champagne while I'm being paid by Moët & Chandon. Personally I think it's high time organisations such as the USDA be held accountable for continuing to issue advice that's harmful to people's health long after it has become clear to bodies such as the Surgeon General's office that there is no evidence to support their advice. As you will learn later in this book, this advice is the main reason that we have a worldwide obesity epidemic on our hands. However, lies aren't new. You were lied to by the US and UK governments about weapons of mass destruction (WMD) in Iraq. Well, you have been lied to again. Dietary animal fat does not cause heart disease. The WMD in your cupboard is not animal fat.

Before explaining what does cause heart disease, let's see why it's important to eat animal fats and why it's dangerous to cut down on them.

BASIC BIOLOGY

I know you did basic biology at school and loved it. I thought so! Don't worry, as this bit of biology is for dummies. Surrounding every cell in your body is a cell membrane that controls what enters and leaves the cell. The cell membrane is composed of fats, including saturated or animal fats, cholesterol and protein. The fats, cholesterol and protein are critical for the functioning of each and every cell in your body.

Inside the cell is the nucleus, which contains your DNA (genes). Surrounding the nucleus is a nuclear membrane, which is also composed of fats and protein. All the internal parts of a cell have a membrane surrounding them, in the same way that each room in your home has walls separating one room from the next. The structure of these membranes is vitally important for the survival of the cell. Figure 3.4 shows a human cell.

Figure 3.4: A human cell

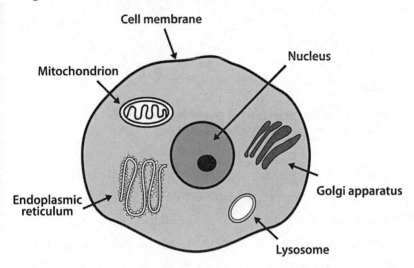

Figure 3.5 shows the cell membrane and all the internal membranes as made up of two layers of fat with various proteins and cholesterol. Much of the fat in these membranes is composed of saturated fat, which is present in dairy produce such as milk, cheese, cream and butter and fat from meats. Animal fat is important because it's solid at room temperature, so it's able to add structure to the membrane. Most other fats are liquid at room temperature and aren't able to support the structure of the membrane. Animal fats give support, rigidity and solidity to all membranes. Without them, the membrane would be a floppy mess.

Figure 3.5: Structure of a cell membrane

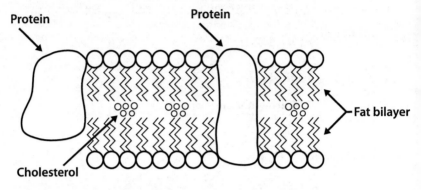

Two layers of fat (fat bilayer) are the basic component.
Protein and cholesterol are also components.

In order to make new cells and repair old ones, animal fat is the single most important part of the diet. Animal fat is even more important for growing children, who are forming millions of new cells. Lowering the animal fat content of the diet of a growing child is very dangerous for a number of reasons; it's essentially guaranteeing illness.

Animal fats are important for other reasons too:

- They are necessary for the absorption of fat-soluble vitamins, such as vitamins A, D and E.
- One of the reasons osteoporosis has become so prevalent is because people have a lower level of vitamin D these days and thus aren't able to absorb calcium in sufficient amounts to sustain well-mineralised bone.
- Animals fed on natural pastures produce lots of conjugated linoleic acid (CLA), an oil that's a proven anti-cancer substance. It's found in high amounts in grass-fed animals such as lambs, sheep, goats and cattle.

There are many compounds in animal produce (and in plants as well) that may be beneficial and that we know little about. There is much to be gained by eating lots of fats: they are the single most important constituent of the diet. Yet the USDA and many other national government agencies in the US and in other countries continue to advise people to cut down on animal fat. Why would they do this? Initially it may have been ignorance, as they were depending on false evidence such as the Seven Countries Study conducted by Professor Ancel Keys. Yet since 1999, when the US Surgeon General's office declared there was no hard evidence linking heart disease and dietary fat, these organisations have persisted with the same message. Why keep supporting a statement when there's no credible evidence to back it up?

The answer would appear to be money. Since the banking crisis that began in 2008, we're all now fully aware that the Western world is based on greed. Multinational food manu-facturers employ many people and pay huge tax revenues, so they can exert a lot of political clout. They have burrowed their way into every government agency responsible for issuing nutritional advice in most of the major economic powers in the world. These companies are major sponsors of most medical conferences dealing with nutrition, national heart associations, national dietetic associations, and indeed any organisation issuing nutritional advice. Let's look at the sponsors of some national dietetic associations as an example, since dieticians are the main professionals offering nutritional advice in our society. Coca-Cola, PepsiCo and GlaxoSmithKline are sponsors (partners) of the American Dietetic Association. Some of their Premium Sponsors include Kellogg's, Mars,

McNeil Nutritionals (makers of Splenda sweetener) and Abbott Nutrition. Kellogg's, Nestlé and Unilever are sponsors of the Dietary Association of Australia, while Kellogg's, Danone and Abbott Nutrition are sponsors of the Irish Dietetic Association. The British Dietetic Association refuses to release the names of its sponsors.

To quieten people opposing their viewpoint, they are now making it illegal in most US states for anyone other than a doctor or dietician to offer nutritional advice. I sense the same companies may have something to do with this.

When food companies reduced or removed fat from our food, it became tasteless and unpalatable. As a result, they decided to replace the fat with sugar. They used sucrose as well as high fructose corn syrup (HFCS). These definitely made the food much tastier, but this has ended up being a major mistake: the introduction of high fructose corn syrup has led to the onset of the obesity epidemic. HFCS was introduced to the food chain in the US in the mid-1970s and a few years later in Europe and other countries worldwide. This resulted in a massive increase in the consumption of sugar, particularly fructose. Because HFCS is dirt cheap, food companies made huge profits and continue to do so at the expense of your health. Since the same companies control the information you receive about food and nutrition, they make sure that the truth about animal fat and about HFCS never sees the light of day. It's only when major investors suggest that they remove the sugar that we now see companies such as Coca-Cola using stevia, which is a natural substance, as a sweetener. Investors know that when the truth emerges about fats and HFCS, these companies will have lawsuits on their hands and as a consequence their shares on the stock market will fall in value. Investors are urging these companies to act quickly to minimise the damage.

I find it remarkable that investors can get these companies to act more responsibly, but governments and world bodies such as the WHO are powerless. You can now understand why I have no faith in what we call Western society: it really is controlled by money. There is no wisdom, no respect for people and no respect for the earth we live on and which feeds us. The economic crisis has shown us how interconnected politics, banking and these food companies are and how they will destroy everything you and I value for their economic gain.

Now for a bit more basic biology.

CHOLESTEROL AND SATURATED FAT

Cholesterol and saturated fat are two very different substances despite the fact that many people confuse the two. For the most part, saturated fat is animal fat, such as cheese, milk, yoghurt, etc. Cholesterol happens to be found in exactly the same foods but is a totally different substance. Figures 3.6a and 3.6b illustrate this point.

Figure 3.6a: Cholesterol

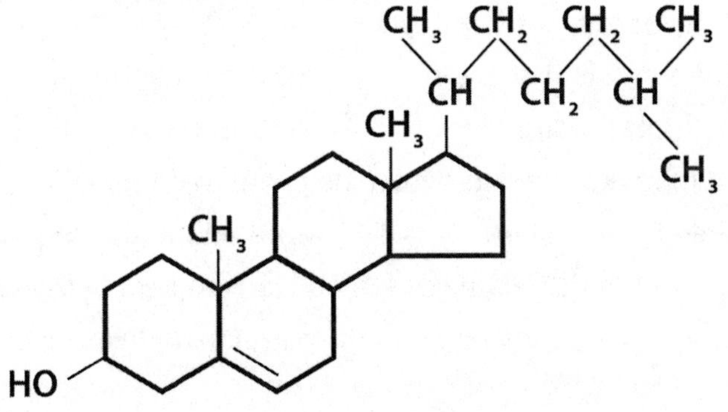

Figure 3.6b: Saturated fat

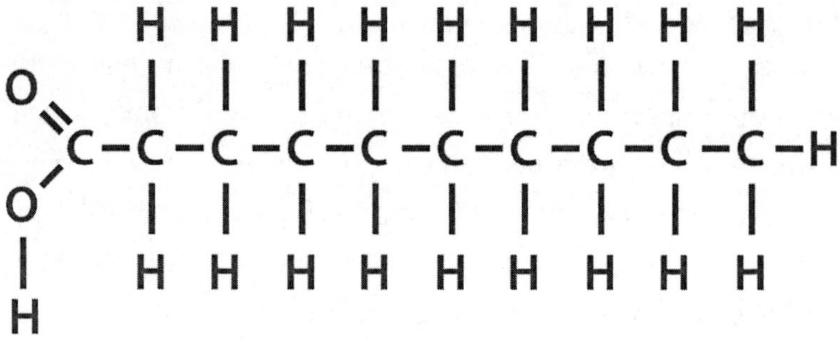

$$O=C-C-C-C-C-C-C-C-C-C-H$$

(structural diagram of a saturated fatty acid: a carboxylic acid group with O double-bonded to C, O–H below, and a chain of ten carbon atoms each bonded to hydrogen atoms above and below)

As you can see, the chemical structure isn't at all similar. Cholesterol is made up of ring structures, whereas saturated fat is a long chain of carbon atoms. Ring structures aren't found in fats. Cholesterol isn't a fat at all! Shocked and confused? I'm sure you are.

Cholesterol is probably the single most important molecule in your body. As you have already learned, it forms part of the cell membrane and other membranes inside the cell. It's particularly important for growing children, but it's also very important for cell replacement and cell repair in adults. It's the major constituent of breast milk. Many hormones in the body are made from cholesterol, including the sex hormones oestrogen, progesterone and testosterone as well as cortisol, which helps you cope with stress.

Cholesterol is also necessary for the manufacture of vitamin D, which plays a number of vital roles. In the liver, cholesterol is used to make bile salts, which help you to digest fats and oils in the diet. Cholesterol acts as an antioxidant and so protects against free radical damage, which leads to heart disease and cancer. Far from causing heart disease, it actually protects you from heart disease – feeling more confused? There's more to come. Cholesterol is also needed for the proper functioning of the central nervous system. Low levels of cholesterol have been linked to depression, suicide and aggressive behaviour. In addition, cholesterol is necessary for the health of the gut wall; low levels have been linked to gut problems such as poor absorption.

As you can see, cholesterol is a mighty important molecule, especially for pregnant women and growing children. This is why many primitive peoples reserve certain foods for pregnant women, such as eggs, the yolk of which is rich in cholesterol. Cholesterol is so important in the body that every cell is able to manufacture it, but 80 per cent is made in the liver and only a small percentage comes from our diet. Knowing this fact alone, you can immediately see the senselessness in reducing dietary cholesterol.

Now comes the really confusing part. Cholesterol is carried from the liver to the various parts of the body where it's needed on a protein called low-density lipoprotein (LDL). You may be familiar with the term 'LDL cholesterol', also called 'bad cholesterol'. LDL is the bus and cholesterol is the passenger, but there are many other passengers on this bus, including all types of fats and fat-soluble vitamins. Why not just call it LDL to stop the confusion – unless, of course, you want to deliberately create confusion?

LDL delivers cholesterol to the cells of the body. Any excess cholesterol not needed is then mopped up and returned to the liver by high-density lipoprotein (HDL), also called 'HDL cholesterol' even though it has little or no cholesterol attached to it.

These terms do nothing for the credibility of science or medicine. All they've achieved is a world of total confusion where we go around using senseless terms. Worse still, everyone thinks dietary fat has everything to do with your LDL level and that if your LDL level is too high, you need to reduce fat in the diet. Nothing could be further from the truth. Professor Ancel Keys, who single-handedly demonised fats, admitted this in 1997. To quote him, 'There is no connection whatsoever between cholesterol in food and cholesterol in blood and we have known that all along' (Keys et al., 1993). Despite this clear and unequivocal statement, we still have government and medical advice saying the opposite. Why are we being misled yet again? I sense another agenda at work here. Could it be the drug companies or the food companies? Or worse still, is it both?

The truth is that your liver controls the level of cholesterol in your body, not your diet. If there's too much cholesterol in your diet, your liver will just make less. In other words, your liver will compensate for your dietary intake. Eat as much cholesterol as you wish.

Enough about cholesterol and fats, let's go back to the food pyramid. In my humble opinion, the advice given in the food pyramid is not only wrong, it's very, very wrong. It's so wrong that I've been forced to create my own food pyramid (Figure 3.7).

Figure 3.7: My food pyramid

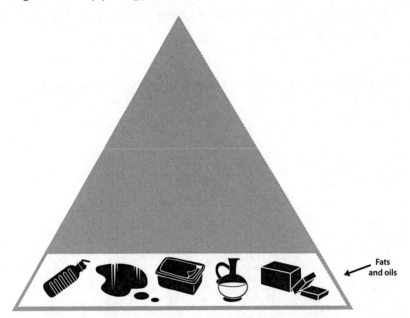

Fats
and oils

The base of the pyramid is now fats and oils because these are the foods you should eat liberally, as they're the most important food group in the diet. This is why primitive peoples such as the Eskimo, Sami and Masai are able to survive and stay so healthy. Fats are a great source of energy as well as all the other benefits mentioned above.

At the top of the pyramid, representing foods you should eat sparingly, I have put carbohydrates, with an additional note to exclude sugar (sucrose and HFCS) completely. There's no problem with a little starch such as potato, but too much is fattening. Many of the primitive peoples I have spent time with consume very little or no starch. Your body can survive by getting all its energy needs from fats. However, if you're an athlete or engaged in physical work every day, such as manual labour, then I suggest you eat lots of carbohydrate, as you'll need it as a quick source of energy. In other words, you'll burn it up and not store it as fat. Figure 3.8 is the pyramid again with carbohydrates (starch and sugar) added.

Figure 3.8: My food pyramid, with carbohydrates added

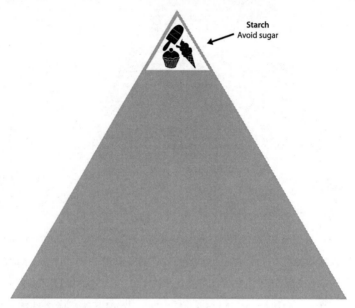

Essentially I've turned the USDA food pyramid on its head. What they have put at the bottom, I've put at the top and vice versa. I have also changed things in the middle of the pyramid.

The second most important food in my pyramid is protein. To build a healthy body, everyone, especially growing children, needs protein. Yet according to the USDA it's less important than fruit and vegetables. Whoever was advising the USDA clearly wasn't a parent feeding a family and clearly had little knowledge of nutrition. Everyone knows the critical importance of protein in the diet, with the exception of the USDA; they prefer to rank fruits and vegetables as more important. The years I spent working in Africa left me in no doubt about the dangers of not eating enough protein. Protein deficiency leads to retarded growth, lethargy, swelling of the legs and abdomen due to oedema, breakdown of the skin and thinning of the hair. These children are more at risk of infection as well. Many die of relatively mild infections, as they have poor immunity. Thus, fats are the most important food and protein ranks second on my pyramid.

Figure 3.9: My food pyramid, with protein and dairy added

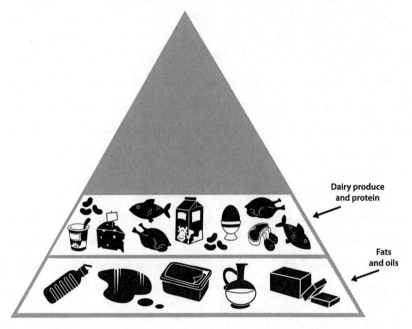

Dairy is a perfect combination of fat and protein, which is why it's regarded as the perfect food and why it's given to babies and young children. I would rank dairy in the same category as protein and so I've placed it at the same level as protein in the pyramid. I am of course referring to real milk, not the stuff found in supermarkets, which is pasteurised and in some cases homogenised and has had much of the fat removed (more about this later in the book).

Since fats and proteins are body-building foods, they occupy the bottom two layers of my pyramid – you should eat lots of these foods. In Nature, fat and protein occur together, as this is what Nature intended you to eat. For example, free-range hen or duck eggs are probably the most complete food available and are rich in fat and protein. An average beefsteak is also about 50 per cent protein and 50 per cent fat.

Fish is also a wonderful combination of fat and protein. The protein in fish is less dense and easier to digest compared to beef. Fish oils are rich in vitamins A, D, E and K. I was given cod liver oil as a child to help the absorption of calcium and phosphorus so that my bones were strong and healthy. To this day I still take cod liver oil intermittently. Fish eggs are especially rich in nutrients and are prized by many cultures as a delicacy.

In Figure 3.10 you'll see that I have added a space for seeds and nuts on my food pyramid. My reason for doing this is because people in the Western world are often deficient in essential oils, especially fish oil and flaxseed oil, both of which contain omega 3. Since seeds and nuts contain a nice mixture of oil and protein, they make a useful snack.

Figure 3.10: My food pyramid, with seeds and nuts

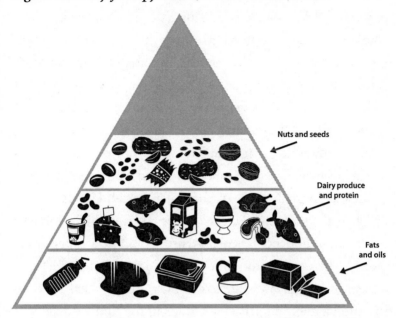

Less important in the diet is fruit and vegetables. Many cultures exist without either fruit or vegetables. For example, the Inuit of northern Canada, the Eskimo of Greenland and the Sami in northern Scandinavia live in latitudes where it's too cold to grow fruit and vegetables. If they have lived for centuries in these environments and remain in good health, we should respect this fact, not ignore it.

Coming back to the food pyramid again, I advise you to eat fruit and vegetables, but I have placed them close to the top of the pyramid, as they are less important. This flies in the face of government advice to eat 'five a day'. I don't know who came up with this slogan, but it has no basis in the world of nutrition.

As mentioned earlier, I'm putting starch (potatoes, rice, pasta, porridge, bread) at the tip of the pyramid, as it's the least important food (except if you exercise or do a lot of physical work). Starch is fine occasionally, especially if it's wholemeal and unrefined. However, it shouldn't be eaten regularly if you're overweight, obese or have diabetes, as starch is just a long chain of glucose molecules and when absorbed will raise your blood sugar level. If you must eat starch, eat it in the middle of the day and use low-glycemic forms of starch, such as brown rice instead of white rice or brown soda bread instead of white rolls, batch loaf or sliced pan.

Sugar, especially table sugar (sucrose) and HFCS, which is labelled as fructose-glucose, corn syrup, high fructose syrup and high fructose corn syrup, should be avoided completely. There is way too much sugar in the Western diet and dangerously high levels since the food industry started adding HFCS to virtually all processed foods in the mid-1970s. If you want to know how damaging sugar is to your health, I suggest you read *Pure, White and Deadly* by Professor John Yudkin. John Yudkin was a professor of physiology who spent his life researching and writing about the effects of high levels of sugar on human physiology. He considered anything over 50 grams of sucrose a day to be very dangerous. Above this level, sugar begins to wreak havoc with liver biochemistry in much the same way that high levels of alcohol does. In 2010 the average person in the Western world was consuming 150 grams of sugar a day.

What you may not know is that sugar is not only the root cause of the obesity epidemic, but is also the root cause of what's referred to as metabolic syndrome, i.e. the disorders that many obese people suffer from, such as diabetes, hypertension, heart disease, gout, raised blood LDL levels and fatty liver. If you want to read more about this you can refer to my e-book, *The Big Fat Secret* (McKenna, 2012).

Figure 3.11: My food pyramid – the full version

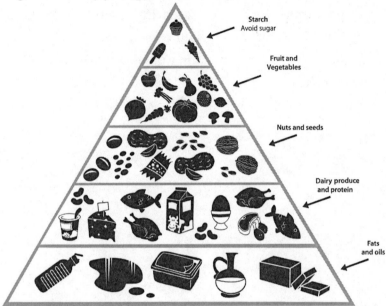

I don't believe it's necessary to tell people how much of each food group one should eat. I have more respect for people and will allow their natural hunger and sense of fullness to control food intake. I was never told how much to eat and I feel certain most of you were never told either. It's true to say that we're in the midst of an obesity epidemic and that people are eating more today. This has to do with the malfunction of the hormone leptin, called leptin resistance, which again is caused by excessively high levels of sugar in the diet. (I explain this in my book on obesity, *The Big Fat Secret* (2012).)

I have now completed my food pyramid. Hopefully it brings some common sense to the discussion about what to eat. I'm trying to balance the misinformation being dished out by government agencies. This misinformation serves only to confuse you and make you increasingly dependent on manu-factured or processed foods. Don't trust any information from politicians, government agencies or any other official body. Trust in Nature and in your own instincts.

In the next chapter I'm going to look at what we call the modern diet.

Chapter 4
Typical Modern Diet

INTRODUCTION

I don't like to bump into my patients in the supermarket, as they become very self-conscious of the contents of their shopping trolley. The feeling is totally mutual, as I don't like people peeking at my basket – I buy as little as possible in the supermarket and so I seldom need a trolley. However, I'm no saint and have weaknesses for certain 'unhealthy' foods (more about my weaknesses later). Examining the contents of people's trolleys is interesting, as they reflect the types of foods being consumed. What's clear from my observations is that people have lost the plot. They no longer know which foods are necessary for good health. This isn't surprising when you see all the conflicting advice and when you're constantly exposed to misleading adverts and are being misled by your government. Worse still, many adverts for sugary snacks and breakfast cereals are being directed at young children. The lack of dietary common sense is reflective of a society that has lost its direction and is essentially in a state of decline.

Did you know that in the Western world, 70 per cent of our diet is now processed foods? Energetically speaking, processed food is dead food: it lacks the natural energy and taste of fresh foods. Processed food is dead food dressed up to look like real food in the same way that one can dress up a corpse to look like it's alive. I'm genuinely at a loss to explain all the harmful effects of eating processed food, but I'll try. I feel particularly sad for the many young children who consume much of this food and may never learn the art of growing, preparing and cooking real food.

A TYPICAL BREAKFAST

I recently spent the weekend at a friend's house and watched what people were eating at breakfast. There were two children and two adults (mom and dad). For all four of them, breakfast began with cereal. One had cornflakes, another had Coco Pops and the other two had Rice Krispies. All four used milk and sugar on their cereal. This was followed by a few slices of toasted white bread with margarine spread and marmalade, along with tea or coffee with milk and sugar added. One of the children took six teaspoons of sugar in her tea. The adults also had orange juice from a carton. They told me that this was what they ate almost every day. To say I was shocked was an understatement. Let's take a closer look at this breakfast.

The cereal

Modern food manufacturing techniques remove most of the nutrients (fibre, vitamins, minerals and enzymes) from the cereal, be it wheat, rice or corn. Artificial chemicals such as colourants, flavourants and sweeteners are added to make the cereal look and taste good. Worse still, sugar is then added to guarantee the product will sell. Essentially, all the goodness is removed, damaging chemicals are added and a highly addictive substance – sugar – is added. This inferior food is then dressed up in a fancy cardboard box with pictures to make it look natural and healthy. There is now evidence that commercial breakfast cereals may be toxic because of damage to the proteins in the cereal during manufacture.

The saying that there is as much nutrition in the cardboard box as in the cereal itself isn't far from the truth. The advertisements suggesting that commercial cereal is enriched with vitamins and minerals are very misleading: the levels of vitamins and minerals added is a small percentage of the recommended daily allowance (RDA). And in any case, the minerals often aren't even well absorbed, as phytic acid in the cereal blocks the absorption of certain minerals in the gut. This is why all natural cereals should be left to soak overnight – in order to lower the level of phytic acid. This is called predigestion of cereals. For example, if you want to eat a healthier, non-processed cereal such as oats for breakfast, it's essential to soak it for at least 8 hours before cooking it. There's little point in soaking processed cereals, as you would be better off not consuming them in the first place.

The milk

This topic always creates a lot of controversy. I'll discuss milk in detail later in the book (see Chapter 6), but I'll quickly mention a few points here.

The best milk is always raw milk, fresh from the animal. In many parts of Europe, including the UK and Ireland, it's possible to buy milk directly from the farmer, provided the dairy herd has been checked for tuberculosis and brucellosis. Most families of dairy farmers use this raw milk themselves, as they don't like the taste of pasteurised milk. Many nations, including France, favour using raw milk to make cheese; they say it's sacrilegious to use pasteurised milk, as all the good bacteria, which are very important in making cheese, have been killed by the process of pasteurisation.

Raw milk is best because it contains lactic acid-producing bacteria that protect against harmful, pathogenic bugs. The process of pasteurisation destroys these bacteria, leaving the finished product devoid of all living bacteria, good or bad. Because it's still a living product, raw milk will sour if left to stand, producing buttermilk. Many cultures use soured milk to replace good bacteria in the body. When you consider that 90 per cent of your body is composed of bacteria (yes, 90 per cent), you can see why it's important to replace these bacteria every day. This is why so many people take soured milk, buttermilk or live yoghurt as often as possible. The Fulani in West Africa used to bring me soured milk every morning (not that I always drank it), while in southern Africa, people drink buttermilk to boost their health.

If pasteurised milk is left to stand, it will putrefy and become toxic – putrefactive chemicals such as putrescine, cadaverine and nervine are quite toxic. Pasteurised milk is a dead product devoid not just of bacteria, but of the enzymes necessary for the proper digestion of milk. This is why so many people have become allergic to milk over the past 50 years. Personally, I believe it's much healthier to use what Nature intended: raw milk.

Most of the milk available in supermarkets is pasteurised and comes in plastic containers. Unfortunately, milk has become big business, where profit is the main concern, not your health. My honest advice is to find an organic farmer close to where you live and buy directly from him or her. Farms that sell directly to the general public have to adhere to higher levels of hygiene than ordinary dairy farms.

Sugar

Sugar and white flour form the foundation of the modern Western diet. Not to put too fine a point on it, but sugar is now increasingly being regarded as a poison. It is unquestionably the single most damaging component of our diet. I say this because it's linked to many degenerative diseases, the so-called diseases of civilisation, which I'll describe shortly. We have known this since Dr Weston Price carried out his studies in the 1930s (see Chapter 2). It was only from experimental studies done in the 1950s and 60s that the biochemistry has been worked out in sufficient detail to label it as a poison. It wreaks havoc with the liver in particular. Yet it's everywhere in the modern diet – in breakfast cereals, soft drinks, fruit juices, sports drinks, cakes and biscuits, but also in virtually all processed foods (tins, bottles, jars and packets). In contrast, it's absent from the diet of primitive peoples. Sugar is the white man's poison.

Prior to the 1800s, there was little sugar in our diet. The production of sugar really began with the growing of sugar cane as a cash crop in North and South America. Sugar cane was grown on huge plantations. The sugar was extracted and then sold commercially. It then began to appear in many different foods and began to appear on the dining table of many homes.

Everyone is intrinsically aware that too much sugar is bad for you. Native Americans warned that it would weaken the body and scientists have been warning for many decades that it's the root cause of many disorders. This wisdom has fallen on deaf ears. Multinational food companies are making huge profits from the sale of processed foods by convincing us that these foods are good for us. These same companies sponsor many prominent scientific and medical organisations. The relationship between governments and the food companies is too cosy. These companies are trying to exert too much influence on politicians, not just in the US, but worldwide. It's no wonder why the truth about sugar is never spoken about.

In 2011, the WHO was preparing to warn people about the dangers of too much sugar in the diet. One member of the US administration in Washington got a call from the CEOs of some of these food manufacturers to ask him to intervene. Within 24 hours he was on a plane to the WHO headquarters in Geneva to warn this so-called independent organisation that their funding would be cut if they didn't take sugar off their agenda. Needless to say, nobody got warned about the dangers of sugar. This was reported in the BBC programme *The Men Who Made Us Fat*, which aired in 2012. This is a scandalous revelation and essentially makes a mockery of the independence of UN organisations.

The food industry is the biggest industry in the US. Its financial clout controls the medical profession, scientists, dieticians, politicians and clearly even the WHO. The food industry will silence anyone who dares to question the role of sugar. However, there are now signs that things are about to change. Investors are worried that as the truth about sugar emerges over the coming months and years, the value of the stock of these companies will fall. Investors are now insisting that sugar be removed from many of these foods. For example, Coca-Cola has already begun to use stevia, a natural sweetener, instead of sugar.

What are the main dangers associated with high levels of sugar in the diet? Let's take a quick look at some of these dangers now. Sugar has many other harmful effects in the body, but the list below should suffice to discourage you from eating it.

Obesity

There is now sufficient experimental and clinical evidence to show that sugar, especially fructose, is responsible for the obesity epidemic. Both table sugar (sucrose) and high fructose corn syrup (HFCS) are composed of glucose and fructose. Glucose is quite safe, but in large amounts fructose is as toxic as alcohol and has almost identical effects on the liver as alcohol. Yet it's freely given to children and even added to infant milk formula. It's wreaking havoc with the health of people across the globe. Nobody in authority is willing to say anything about this out of fear. They have been effectively gagged by the food companies. The volume of research supporting the role of fructose in the obesity epidemic is now so overwhelming that some doctors are speaking out. I suspect that soon there will be a lot of heads rolling.

Heart disease

By heart disease, I'm referring to coronary artery disease, or blocked arteries, as it's popularly known. There is now a wealth of evidence linking sugar with this disease. Heart disease doesn't exist among primitive peoples, but as soon as these people start to eat modern foods, they begin to develop heart disease. Researchers such as Alfredo Lopez (1966) and Edward Ahrens (1986) repeatedly demonstrated a link between sugar and coronary artery disease. However, their work, like that of Professor John Yudkin, has been largely ignored, as it conflicts with government agencies. If the public were made aware of this link and were advised to cut sugar out of the diet, the powerful food companies would be reduced to midgets and tax returns would shrink accordingly. The food manufacturers need sugar to sell their food.

Diabetes

Everyone is aware of the link between diabetes and sugar. Yet despite all the medical and scientific knowledge, some spokespeople for the food industry are now suggesting that there's no link at all. What an insult to our intelligence! The strategy seems to be to create controversy and delay the inevitable. The tobacco industry did exactly the same thing back in the 1970s.

Raised cholesterol

This should be called raised LDL (low-density lipoprotein), the so-called bad cholesterol. The main reason why your LDL rises is because of sugar ingestion. Professor Yudkin and Professor Ahrens demonstrated this in their research. More recently, Professor Richard Johnson et al. (2007) demonstrated the mechanism by which sugar causes a range of metabolic disorders, including raised LDL, raised triglycerides and increased stickiness of blood platelets.

Fatty liver

Sugar is a combination of two simple sugars joined together, which is broken down in the gut to glucose and fructose. It's the fructose part that's responsible for many of the damaging effects of sugar. Most of the fructose is converted to fat in the liver, whereas very little of the glucose ends up as fat – it's burned off for energy. Nature didn't intend for us to eat lots of fructose, but *did* intend for us to eat moderate amounts of glucose, which is found in starchy foods such as potatoes, rice and porridge. The glucose component of sugar is relatively safe, but the fructose component is deadly. Much of the fat produced by the metabolism of fructose enters the blood, but some is stored in the liver and ends up causing fatty liver. Alcohol is metabolised in the liver in almost exactly the same way.

Abnormal bacterial flora

Sugar promotes the growth of bad bacteria in the gut. It also promotes the overgrowth of some good microbes, such as *Candida albicans*, resulting in a condition called dysbiosis. I discuss this condition in detail in my book *Hard to Stomach* (2002).

Cancer

A high sugar intake in the diet is positively associated with cancer in both laboratory animals and in humans. Cancer cells require a huge amount of energy in the form of sugar to grow and multiply. This may partly explain why cancer is so common amongst Westerners and so uncommon amongst people eating a natural, unprocessed diet.

Ageing

Sugar causes wrinkles in the skin. It's now known that sugar attaches to the protein molecules in the skin (collagen and elastin) to form harmful new molecules called advanced glycation end products (AGEs). This may be why diabetics age so much faster than non-diabetics.

In the 1990s, a low-calorie diet was shown to delay the ageing process by switching off the ageing genes and turning on the genes that keep you looking young. A low-calorie diet has also been shown to prolong life in both animals and humans.

White bread

White bread is mostly made from refined wheat flour. Whole wheat contains starch, protein, fibre, vitamins, minerals and enzymes. Refined wheat contains starch and protein that has been chemically treated but lacks the enzymes, vitamins and minerals that help your body to digest the wheat. Digestion of refined wheat calls on your body's own reserves of enzymes, vitamins and minerals. For example, B vitamins are essential for the metabolism of wheat, but the B vitamins are removed in the refining process. Thus, if your body doesn't have enough B vitamins, you won't be able to metabolise the wheat and get energy from it. Refined foods are not only depleted foods, but they can end up robbing you of your reserves of vitamins, minerals and enzymes. In other words, they place a burden on your body.

Margarine spread

These spreads contain harmful trans fats, which are known to cause many health problems. If you know a little bit about how they're made, you might not be so eager to use them and will opt for real butter instead. Here are the essential steps for how to make easy-to-spread margarine:

1. The cheapest oils (corn, canola, soya) are extracted and allowed to go rancid.
2. These oils are then mixed with metal particles, usually nickel and aluminium.
3. The oil and metal mixture is then subjected to hydrogen gas at high temperature and high pressure.
4. Emulsifiers and starch are added to the mixture to make it more solid.
5. The mixture is again subjected to high temperature to remove bad odours.
6. The mixture is bleached to remove the grey colour.
7. Artificial colourants and flavourants are added to make it look and taste like butter.
8. It's then compressed and packed into plastic tubs.

Worse still, it's even endorsed by some national heart associations. My honest advice is to avoid these margarine spreads like the plague. A nickel catalyst used in the production of margarine called Raney nickel is actually 50 per cent nickel and 50 per cent aluminium. Some of the metal particles remain in the finished product and are eaten by people. Aluminium is associated with Alzheimer's disease and with osteoporosis and may even be associated with the development of cancer cells. Nickel is a metal that increases your sensitivity to your environment. In other words, you begin to develop allergic reactions to things you were tolerant of before.

As regards trans fats, suffice it to say that the Dutch government was so concerned about the negative effects of trans fats that they banned the sale of margarine containing trans fats. Trans fats block the essential fatty acid linoleic acid, which is a natural beneficial fat for the body. Trans fats also raise blood LDL levels and triglyceride levels, both of which are associated with heart disease. Not only do trans fats have detrimental effects on the cardiovascular system, but they can also damage the reproductive system by decreasing testosterone and increasing abnormal sperm counts as well as interfering with pregnancy and lowering the quality of breast milk. They can also affect your immune system by lowering the effectiveness of certain immune responses (e.g. B cell response, which enables you to make antibodies). They also interfere with the liver's ability to metabolise toxins and carcinogens. These are only some of the side effects of trans fats. Now you have an idea why the Dutch government banned them.

My advice to you is to avoid all margarines, spreads and shortenings. Use butter, which is 100 per cent pure and natural. Try to buy the butter of cattle fed on natural pastures, as it's richer in nutrients and is usually yellower in colour. Alternatively, buy New Zealand butter, which comes from grass-fed animals.

Jams and marmalades

If the jam or marmalade is made from fruit and fruit only and no sugar has been added, then it's safe to use in small amounts. However, most commercial and some homemade jams and marmalades are laden with sugar (sucrose) and so are best avoided. Honey is preferable, but use natural honey, not the commercial honey available in supermarkets (with the exception of manuka honey from New Zealand, which is well known at this stage for its health-giving properties).

Tea and coffee

Tea and coffee both contain caffeine and theobromine, which stimulate the adrenal glands to produce adrenalin. This in turn causes the liver to release glucose into the bloodstream. The sugar is then converted to energy, which gives you the lift or kick you get from stimulant drinks such as tea and coffee. Too much caffeine day after day ultimately exhausts the adrenal glands, so you aren't able to boost your energy levels and may eventually end up with chronic fatigue. Caffeine can also irritate the lining of the stomach, causing increased acidity, and can interfere with normal sleep patterns and ultimately cause insomnia.

If you want to do yourself and your family a big favour, switch to green tea. It's so beneficial to your health that it is the subject of a lot of medical and scientific research. It's full of antioxidants that protect against degenerative diseases such as osteoarthritis, heart disease and cancer. The plant originates in China, where people drink many cups a day. The tea is made from the leaves of the plant. It has been shown to have anti-cancer properties, which may explain why the Chinese have such a low lung cancer rate despite the fact that they smoke so heavily. Studies done at the University of Edinburgh (Gaskell, 2013) showed that green tea reduced blood pressure, reduced blood LDL levels, reduced body fat and reduced body weight. Studies done at the Linus Pauling Institute at Oregon State University (University of Maryland

Medical Center, nd), showed that green tea was able to enhance the immune system and was able to suppress auto-immune disorders such as rheumatoid arthritis. Green tea has also been shown to protect against a number of cancers, notably breast and colon cancer. This is a tea well worth using every day of your life. Its benefits are legendary and the research supports this. It's available in most health food shops and many supermarkets. Try to buy the loose leaves, not the green tea bags.

Fruit juice

Commercial fruit juices from the supermarket are essentially coloured water. They have no nutritional value whatsoever. Most commercial fruit juices have a negative nutritional value in that they often contain sugar and artificial additives. Avoid them if you can – buy fresh fruit and make your own juice at home. It's an excellent idea to buy a good juicer and involve the whole family in making their own mixtures of vegetable and fruit juices. Alternatively, just drink water.

Now that I have ruined your favourite breakfast, I'll offer healthy alternatives in the next chapter. But the ruination doesn't stop with breakfast. I shall now do a hatchet job on lunch and supper as well so that you are left in no doubt about the effects of modern foodstuffs on human health. The purpose of this exercise is to wake you up from deep slumber and get your body functioning well so that you can enjoy this experience called life.

Let's now take a quick look at a typical lunch in modern Europe.

LUNCH

A typical adult lunch, especially in times of recession, may consist of a hamburger and chips or a sandwich with either a soft drink or a fruit juice. Alternatively, it may consist of pizza and chips or some other starchy food with a bit of protein. From observing people at lunch in the city, it seems that many view lunch as a chance to stock up on calories, hence the emphasis on starchy, filling foods.

It's interesting to note that starch is indeed filling, but only temporarily. Protein is much more filling, as it takes the stomach much longer to digest protein. The best combination for filling your stomach is protein and animal fat, and fortunately the two often come together. A hamburger is a good idea, provided the quality of the meat is good and provided it's 100 per cent beef with no additives. Most commercial hamburgers are of poor-quality beef and contain less than 50 per cent beef, and so have many additives and don't create that full feeling. Most fast food restaurants will put the hamburger in a bun that's composed of white processed bread, which I have discussed earlier. White processed bread is devoid of many important nutrients such as fibre, enzymes, vitamins and minerals and so can be hard to digest and may end up causing you tummy problems. Hamburger buns are manufactured with two aims in mind: a long shelf life and taste. Firstly, the fibre is removed so that the bun has a long shelf life and can be exported. Secondly, the fibre is replaced with sugar to make the bun taste good. Essentially, fibre, which is good for you, has been removed and has been replaced with an extremely damaging substance: sugar.

Food companies aren't interested in your health or your

welfare. They produce cheap food, dress it up to look like real food or use enticing adverts and sell it for a profit. By adding sugar, which is known to be an addictive substance, they guarantee that you'll come back again and again. Food manufacturers know a lot about making money but little or nothing about nutrition.

Cooking oil

Chips and other foods are often cooked by frying them in vegetable oil, such as sunflower oil. When you heat an oil, you change the chemical structure of the oil and can render the oil harmful to the body. If low heat is used this isn't usually a problem, but if you wish to use high heat, use animal fat such as lard or butter, which is more heat resistant.

Most fast food outlets use vegetable oil at high heat. When this oil is heated and then reheated again and again, it's essentially becoming more and more toxic. When you're young your liver can handle toxicity better, but as you grow older this isn't the case, as liver function slows down, making it more difficult to eliminate toxic chemicals in food. My advice is to avoid all fried foods unless you're the one preparing the food. Ban deep-fat fryers from your kitchen, as they create a hidden source of toxicity for your family. Use only animal fat for high-heat cooking and extra virgin olive oil for low-heat cooking.

So a hamburger and chips may seem like a good idea, as it's cheap, convenient and fast to produce, but you would be better off having a bowl of soup and brown bread or a sandwich made with brown bread and butter and some form of protein, e.g. chicken or ham, in the middle. A hard-boiled egg is the best nutrition you can get, as it's a wonderful combination of protein and fat. Alternatively, have a salad with fresh vegetables and a form of protein such as fish or chicken. For dessert, have fresh fruit or live yoghurt (without sugar). Drink lots of green tea.

The problem with good food is that it takes time to prepare and isn't cheap. However, it's a bit masochistic to continue to damage your body with cheap fast food. When people are pressed for time and money, the fast food option does seem attractive, but you need to be aware that speed and cost aren't factors to take into account when feeding your body. Nutritional value is the only factor to consider.

Lunchboxes

Children's lunchboxes are a real eye-opener. I was shocked when I returned home from Africa and saw the foods that children were eating for break. One word summarises the contents of a typical school lunchbox: sugar! Chocolate bars, cereal bars, sports bars, fizzy drinks, sports drinks, sweets, etc. In the Western world, children seem to get a sugar fix at breakfast, another at the mid-morning break, then again at lunch and sometimes again after school. We're raising a generation of sugar addicts. Wittingly or unwittingly, we're supporting their habit. This is an area where the school could take control and ban all sugary snacks from the premises. Schools where vending machines have been banned have seen a reduction in the body weight of children.

EVENING MEAL

Having raised three children as a single parent, I understand the temptation of using fast food or ready-made meals. I've done it out of desperation. However, evening time is probably the only time of day when the family can be together. It's a chance for everyone to chip in with the task of making a healthy meal. It's a time when children will learn lessons that will dictate their eating pattern for the rest of their lives.

Teach them how to make a simple cooked meal containing protein, starch and vegetables. Educate them about how to select the best produce when shopping for this meal and how to cook the food to get the maximum nutrition from it. It's also a good time to teach them how to bake, especially baking bread.

The preparation of food for your loved ones has a much deeper meaning. It strengthens the bonds between you and your family. Sharing food together is a profound experience and connects you not just physically in the act of sharing food, but also emotionally, in that it's a warm, comforting experience, and spiritually, in that it shows the love you have for them because you have gone to great lengths to feed them healthy food. It also connects all of you with Nature, provided the food is natural and not processed by food companies. This connection with Nature is very important for children to learn about, as Nature is there to help you remain healthy; clearly, food companies are not.

The evening meal is particularly important because it's often the only time of the day when the family can relax and enjoy a meal, as breakfast is usually a rushed affair in the modern world. It's important not to rush the evening meal because of homework or because you want to watch a television programme. The most special time of the day for the modern family is coming together for the evening meal to share not just food, but stories about each person's day, etc. This is the time when parents will learn most about their children and children will learn most about their parents. To rush the experience or to serve takeaways or ready-made meals belittles the experience. This is a golden opportunity for everyone to add their bit of effort or knowledge to the preparation of the healthiest meal possible for you as a family. When everyone is involved it becomes a special event that will linger long in the memory. It's the greatest legacy you can leave your children, as they will learn how to feed themselves well and will nourish their family in turn.

When something is prepared by dedicating a lot of mental focus and physical effort, you're showing respect for the nourishment of your family. When you use natural food you're showing respect for Nature and confirming the fact that you're part of Nature. You're also showing self-respect. By setting high standards for your family, you're guaranteeing their continued health and happiness.

If the evening meal has been a nutritious meal, people will be less inclined to eat sugary snacks afterwards. Their tummies will be full and they won't need to eat again until the following morning. Poor-quality meals such as takeaways often don't satisfy you sufficiently for long, so you tend to indulge in 'grazing', where you munch your way through the cupboards and fridge. People will even eat soil to try to satisfy their craving. The medical term for eating soil is 'pica' and it usually indicates a deficiency of minerals in the body, which can be got from the soil. The mineral content of soil is so important in some cultures that a little bit of soil is added to food before eating it. I have seen this being done in a number of countries, especially in Africa. In Europe, the healing properties of clay have also long been recognised.

Become more aware of the food that you're eating and that you're feeding your family. Ask lots of questions at your supermarket, butcher, greengrocer and baker and demand the best possible. The more you question everything in your society, the more others will do the same. The more we demand real food, the more likely we are to get it. Begin today.

Chapter 5
A Healthy Diet

INTRODUCTION

There is much confusion today about what constitutes a healthy diet. There was little or no confusion 100 years ago or even 50 years ago. Everyone knew which foods were important for good health. What has happened to create such confusion? Where have things gone wrong? I'll answer this shortly, but first let's see if we can define what a healthy diet consists of. It's actually quite simple but requires a bit of explanation.

WATER

Firstly, you have to ask yourself what your body is made up of. If 50 to 60 per cent of the body is water, then this takes precedence over any other food. The interior of a cell is mostly water, the cells of the body are bathed in tissue fluid, which is mostly water, and blood is mostly water as well. In other words, you are mostly water. The quality of this water dictates how efficiently your body will function. The purer the water, the easier it is for your body to use. The purity of your drinking water has become a big issue today and most people are aware that their tap water is simply not up to scratch.

The purity of your water can be tested using a very simple device called a TDS meter. TDS stands for total dissolved solids, or the amount of solid matter hidden in the water. It's a small hand-held device with two metal probes at one end. It's worth investing in a TDS meter. They cost about €20 and can be used for testing all sources of water, such as well water, river water, tap water and bottled waters. You simply place the metal probes in a water sample, press a button on the meter and it displays a digital reading (in parts per million). Pure water will give a reading of zero or very close to zero. Tap water usually has a reading of 450 to 500 parts per million (ppm). Bottled waters vary a lot, between 150 and 500 ppm. The best waters have a reading below 150 ppm and this is what you're aiming for. This means there is less dissolved matter in the water.

The best water on the planet is glacial water from melting glaciers in Pakistan, Scandinavia, Tibet and Chile/Argentina as well as water from artesian wells, e.g. Spa mineral water from Belgium, which is available in all the supermarkets in the UK but not in Ireland. This mineral water has won many awards over the years.

Water is an almost magical substance. When planet Earth was first formed, there was no water on it. It was a dead place with no life. At some point in its history, one or more comets must have collided with it, as comets are mostly frozen water. Today the surface of the planet is mostly water. The presence of water allowed life to begin. What's strange about water is that it doesn't obey the laws of physics. In other words, it doesn't do what all other substances do. For example, when a liquid substance is cooled it changes from a liquid state to a solid state, which means that the atoms in the substance come closer together and are more densely packed, which makes the substance denser. Water in the solid state (ice) should therefore sink if added to a liquid, as all other substances do. Instead, water becomes less dense and floats on top. This allows ice to float on the top of a lake.

Water is also very strange at a molecular level. The water molecule is so amazing that it can mimic the electronic structure of any substance – say, orange juice – it's mixed with. In fact, it starts to behave like this substance if enough of the water molecules adopt the electronic structure of the orange juice. This is the basis for homeopathic medicine.

Water is indeed a very magical substance, and since we're composed mostly of water, we too are magical. The level of purity of the water you drink is important, but the electronic structure of this water is just as important – in other words, what the water has been mixed with. If it has run through pipes and machines, as in the case of tap water, avoid it, as it may well have an undesirable structure. If it has come from a stream, river, underground source or glacier, then the structure is likely to be more natural and so more bio-available, i.e. easier for the body to use. This is the main disagreement that I have with the purification of tap water using various filters such as reverse osmosis filters. Yes, your water will be more pure with the use of a filter, but the structure of the water is not necessarily improved. Water directly from Nature is still the best.

I'll discuss water in a bit more detail later in this book. For now, just keep in mind that it is the single most important nutrient by far.

GOOD BACTERIA

Ninety per cent of the rest of your body is made up of bacteria (shock horror) – yes, bacteria, those things you would rather not see or talk about. Most bacteria are important for human health; very few are harmful (maybe they're not so bad after all). That means that the remaining 10 per cent of your body is human cells.

Almost every culture on this planet replaces the good bacteria every day, either with soured milk, buttermilk or live yoghurt. When raw milk is left to stand or used to make yoghurt, the living bacteria in the milk (lactic acid bacteria) multiply and curd the milk. This is why buttermilk, soured milk products and live yoghurt are so important in the diet – in fact, they're the second most important constituent of a healthy diet after water. Pasteurised milk doesn't have living bacteria in it and so is useless for replacing good bacteria.

I see very few people in the Western world using live cultures as part of their diet. Virtually all the milk products used by people in Europe and North America are made from heat-treated milk (i.e. pasteurised milk). Some people take a probiotic culture bought from a health shop or chemist, which is excellent. If, like most people, you don't have access to live cultures in milk products, then use a probiotic capsule or powder. The best on the market is OptiBac Probiotics, as their product formulations are excellent and are based on sound medical research. Some commercial yoghurts have live cultures but also have sugar added, which is harmful, as you learned in Chapter 4. It's best to avoid such yoghurts and don't give them to children, especially young children; the younger the child, the greater the tendency to become addicted to sugar. The best solution is to make your own yoghurt, which is incredibly simple. Rather than explaining it in words, log on to YouTube and learn, then teach your children how to do it.

All surfaces of the body have a thick coating of bacteria. These surfaces include the skin, the respiratory tract (nose to lungs), the digestive tract all the way from the mouth to the anus, the vagina in females and the urethra in both males and females. You can't see these bacteria, as they are microscopic in size. There are no less than 90 trillion bacteria on your body. We are basically a bacterial colony, with only 10 trillion human cells; hence, we are composed of many more bacterial cells than human cells – nine times more, to be exact.

These bacteria are so important that your body simply would not function without them. They are unseen and unsung heroes. They act as an interface between you and the environment in which you live. They exist to serve you in amazing ways. They are the single most important defence against foreign microbes such as bad bacteria, against viruses and against other invaders.

The gut bacteria in particular are an integral part of your immune system. These wonderful little bacteria supply you with a range of vitamins, including some B vitamins (B1, B2, B5 and B6) and vitamin K, which is important in blood clotting. Recent research (Hamilton, 1999) suggests that the gut flora may actually produce many more micronutrients than previously thought. The gut flora aids all aspects of gut function, mainly by regulating the acid–alkaline balance in different parts of the gut. They also assist with bowel function such that when the colonic flora goes out of balance, constipation or diarrhoea results.

The flora in the colon does something else that is quite amazing. They are able to digest some of the fibre in foods such as beans, lentils and legumes and convert the fibre into short chain fatty acids (SCFAS), which have amazing benefits for you. These acids are called acetic, propionic, butyric, lactic, hippuric and orotic acid. The most important of these is probably butyric acid, which forms the main food for the cells that line the colon. Without sufficient butyric acid the lining of the colon becomes inflamed and colitis, also called ulcerative colitis, begins. A disturbance in the bacterial flora in the gut is now known to play a major role in the onset of colitis. As a consequence, most good gastroenterologists now prescribe probiotics for patients with this condition. Butyric acid is also known to be a key substance in the prevention of colonic cancer and possibly other cancers as well, such as breast, prostate and liver cancer.

A number of these SCFAS, especially acetic and lactic acid, combine to produce an acidic environment, which inhibits nasty pathogens such as typhoid bacteria. These SCFAS inhibit the growth not only of outside invaders, but they also help to prevent normal constituents of the gut flora, such as *Candida albicans*, from overgrowing.

When travelling to a foreign country, take lots of good bacteria in the form of probiotic capsules to prevent traveller's diarrhoea (the OptiBac Probiotics supplement 'For travelling abroad' is good). Also, if you're going to an area of the world where typhoid, cholera or dysentery may be present, it's really important to protect yourself with regular probiotic supplementation. The main problem when travelling is that the probiotic capsules need to be kept refrigerated, so bring a cooler bag.

The benefits of these microscopic creatures are astounding and their effects are felt far beyond the gut. For example, propionic acid helps balance hormonal levels via its effects on the liver. These bacteria have widespread positive effects on virtually all aspects of body function. They co-operate with you and live in harmony with you and ensure you remain healthy. To then go and damage them by using antibiotics unnecessarily or by consuming artificial sweeteners, both of which are known to disturb the flora, is really a shame. This is one reason why I wrote my first book, *Natural Alternatives to Antibiotics* (McKenna, 1996), as I was shocked by the blatant abuse of antibiotics by doctors.

I cannot overstate the importance of the bacterial flora in human health. If you do nothing that I suggest in this book other than take good bacteria every day, you will have helped yourself enormously.

FATS AND PROTEIN

The rest of your body is mainly made up of fats and proteins. Let me explain this. Every cell in your body has a cell membrane around it, which controls what enters and leaves the cell. The cell membrane is made up mostly of fat (phospholipid bilayer, to give it its technical name), with protein and cholesterol scattered throughout. If you look at Figure 5.1, you'll see a drawing of a cell membrane that is composed of an outer layer of fat and an inner layer of fat, hence the term lipid bilayer. You'll also see that this bilayer has proteins embedded in it. These proteins serve to regulate the transport of substances into and out of the cell as well as transmit messages to the cell. Cholesterol forms the third component of all membranes. Thus, the major part of the cell membrane is made up of fat. This is why fat is so important in the diet.

Figure 5.1: *Structure of a cell membrane*

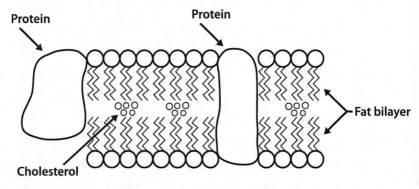

Two layers of fat (fat bilayer) are the basic component.
Protein and cholesterol are also components.

There are many structures inside the cell, such as the nucleus, which contains the DNA or genetic material, and the mitochondria, which releases energy from food. Each of these structures has its own membrane, which is also made up mostly of fat and protein as well as cholesterol. There are many membranes inside the cell, each of them made up of the same building blocks.

A good analogy would be a house that is made up of exterior walls (the cell membrane) and interior walls that divide the house into rooms, each with its own function (the sub-cellular structures). However, the exterior walls may be made of bricks or blocks and the internal walls can be made of a different material, such as plasterboard; this is not true regarding cells, where all the membranes are made of the same material – a fat bilayer, protein and cholesterol.

Cells are grouped together to form tissues with a special function, e.g. muscle tissue, and tissues are grouped together to form organs. Your whole body is primarily composed of fat, then protein and then cholesterol. It's easy, then, to understand that fat, protein and cholesterol are the three most important components of our diet after water and live bacteria.

When I was growing up my mother and grandmother knew this, as did everyone else's mother and granny. All cultures on this planet know that fat and protein (and cholesterol) are vital for survival. Some primitive peoples, such as the Eskimo, eat little else. They survive on fat combined with protein. Cholesterol is found in the same foods as animal fat. Then along came Western scientists who decided they knew better. They decided to reduce the fat in our diet and to demonise the most important type of fat: animal fat such as butter, cheese, milk, etc. Science was the god of truth and issued words of warning that fat in the diet was causing heart disease. Unfortunately, politicians listened to this message and even set up a Senate committee in the US to investigate it. The result was the greatest lie I have ever heard spoken. There is absolutely no evidence linking heart disease with dietary fat. That might shock you, and so it should. Effectively, you have been lied to for over 30 years.

Because of public outcries by scientists and doctors back in the early 1980s and because of four large studies from different countries that effectively disproved the fat–heart disease link, in 1989 the US government asked the Surgeon General's office to produce evidence linking animal fat in the diet with heart disease. They could not produce the evidence and it took no less than 11 years to state this; it was only in 1999, long after the message had been ingrained in everyone's brain, that they agreed there was no evidence.

There are a huge number of scandals within this whole issue. For example, why did it take 11 years to look at the evidence, when you or I could do it within a few days on the internet? Why did a government (the US and the UK governments in particular) tell its people that there was no hard scientific evidence? Why has nobody acknowledged the lie until today and why have no heads rolled? It's a scandal of huge proportion – it has affected the whole world. To this day, doctors are still telling people to reduce animal fats if a patient has heart disease. No wonder there is such confusion. Common sense has been tossed out the window in favour of lies perpetrated by the US and UK governments. It's not the first time that these two governments have co-operated in lying to the general public.

Let's get back to the topic of healthy food. Fat, protein and cholesterol are the building blocks of your body, the foundation stones for good health. They are therefore critically important for a growing child, who is forming new cells all the time. They are important for adults too, as they are needed to repair and replace old cells. Since all the membranes in a cell are mostly made of fat, this constitutes the single most important food group to eat every day.

Let's now look at fats in a bit more detail.

FATS

The study of fats is quite confusing, with complicated terms such as saturated fat, monounsaturated fat, polyunsaturated fat, trans fat, omega 3 and omega 6 fats to name just a few. It's bamboozling! You need to have a degree in chemistry or biochemistry to understand it all. Assuming you don't have a degree in either of these subjects, I'll explain them as simply as possible.

Saturated fats are found in animal fats for the most part and in some tropical oils, such as coconut oil. They tend to be solid or semi-solid at room temperature, e.g. butter. This solidity helps to add shape and structure to all membranes, giving them the necessary stiffness and integrity. Therefore, most of the fat in a membrane is composed of saturated fat. (I'll use the terms 'saturated fat' and 'animal fat' to mean the same thing, as I don't live in the tropics.) The body regards saturated fats as essential and goes to the trouble of making them if you don't eat enough in your diet. The body has a clever way of making them from carbohydrates. (The working of the body and of Nature as a whole is simply amazing.) In my opinion, saturated or animal fat is the single most important part of a healthy diet (after water and bacteria, of course). Here are my reasons for saying this:

- Saturated fats are vital for the structure and function of all cells.
- Saturated fats are important for the absorption of the fat-soluble vitamins A, D, E and K.
- Saturated fats protect against heart disease by lowering

a substance in the bloodstream called Lp(a), which is an indicator of susceptibility to blocked arteries.

- Saturated fats protect your liver from toxins such as alcohol.
- Saturated fats boost the immune system.
- Some saturated fats have antimicrobial properties by protecting against harmful microbes in the gut.
- Saturated fats are quite stable and so do not turn rancid easily. They are useful in cooking and baking.

Unsaturated fats are divided up into monounsaturated and polyunsaturated fats. Monounsaturated fat is the most like saturated fat, as it's chemically quite similar – it has only one double bond, while saturated fat has no double bonds. (Don't worry if you don't understand what a double bond is.) Your body can convert a saturated fat into a monounsaturated fat. A good example of a monounsaturated fat is olive oil, but it's also found in certain nuts, such as almonds, pecans, cashews and peanuts, and in avocados. Like saturated fats, monounsaturated fats are quite stable, do not go rancid easily and can be used in cooking.

Polyunsaturated fats have two or more double bonds and so are quite different from saturated fats. These can't be made by the body, so they are called essential fats – they must be obtained from the diet. Polyunsaturated fats include omega 6 and omega 3 oils, which you probably have heard about already. The two polyunsaturated fats found most commonly in our diet are linoleic acid (omega 6) and linolenic acid (omega 3). Linoleic acid, or omega 6, is found in many vegetable oils, such as sunflower, sesame and evening primrose oils.

Linolenic acid, or omega 3, is found in fish oil and flaxseed oil. Polyunsaturated fats or oils are quite different in that they are liquid at room temperature and turn rancid very quickly, especially linolenic acid (omega 3). They should never be heated or used in cooking.

All fats found in Nature are a combination of saturated and unsaturated fats. For example, olive oil is 75 per cent monounsaturated, 13 per cent saturated and 12 per cent polyunsaturated. Lard or pork fat is 48 per cent monounsaturated, 40 per cent saturated and 12 per cent polyunsaturated. The amounts of omega 3 and omega 6 in animal fat will vary with the diet of the animal.

All forms of fat are essential for good health. Having tested many people over the years, what is obvious is the very low levels of omega 3, or linolenic acid, in the diet of Westerners. I highly recommend a lot of fish oil and flaxseeds (also called linseeds) in the diet to compensate for a possible shortage. In fact, most of my patients already use flaxseed, as it's also a bulking agent to help clear the bowels and I recommend it when treating a digestive problem. I have also recently started asking them to increase the amount of animal fat in the diet to compensate for the misinformation being given by the health authorities.

Fats and proteins tend to occur together in Nature. For example, milk is rich in protein but also has a full complement of fats. Eggs are probably the best food on the planet – they are the most complete food of all, in that they have a wonderful combination of fat and protein. Breast milk is yet another example. Fat and protein are buddies because they form the cell membranes of all living creatures on the planet.

They are inseparable, or so it seems. Interestingly, the third component of cell membranes – cholesterol – is found in the same foods as fats and protein. All three are like the three musketeers.

PROTEIN

Now let's take a close look at protein. After water, good bacteria and fat, protein forms the fourth important part of a healthy diet. It's often written in school books and university textbooks that protein is the most important part of the diet, but this is simply not true. Proteins are also described as the building blocks of the body, and this is also untrue. Protein does assist in the structure of membranes, muscle tissue and other tissues, but the image of protein as the sole building block is misleading. If we use the analogy of the walls of a house, the bricks represent the fat bilayer and the mortar represents the protein, but both are necessary to form a solid structure.

There are many types of protein playing many different roles in the body: structural proteins, which form part of the cell membrane; enzymes, which speed up chemical reactions; hormones, which control chemical reactions and other body functions; and antibodies, which form part of the immune defence. All proteins consist of a long chain of amino acids. There are 22 different amino acids and the body needs all 22 to build the huge array of proteins needed for a healthy body. Your body can actually manufacture some of these amino acids; it can make 14 of the 22. The body can't make the remaining eight amino acids, so these have to be obtained from the diet.

If the protein you consume as food contains all 22 amino acids, it's called a complete protein. Complete proteins are therefore the best form of protein to eat and come from animal sources such as meat, poultry, eggs, dairy produce, fish and shellfish.

If one or more of the 22 amino acids is missing, the protein is referred to as incomplete. Plant proteins such as wheat are generally incomplete. Incomplete protein includes such food as grains, pulses, nuts and vegetables. However, by combining plant proteins such as pulses and grains, it's possible to supply the body with a full complement of amino acids. This is why vegetarians have to carefully mix their foods so as not to become deficient.

Primitive peoples around the world thrived for centuries and many still thrive today on a diet composed mainly of protein and fat with occasional fruits, seeds and nuts. Studies done on these people testify to their high level of health. The fat and protein are invariably animal in origin. However, there are people who also have a very high level of health on a purely plant-based diet. What nobody disagrees about is the very low level of health of people on a diet containing mostly processed foods. This is the worst diet for many reasons. For toxicity reasons (which I made you aware of in Chapter 4), a Western diet causes serious problems. However, what I haven't mentioned yet is the genetic reason. Genetically we have greatest difficulty with cereals and processed milk and with the array of chemicals added to foods. Like many of the primitive cultures on the planet, we have survived mainly on animal produce for centuries. It is only more recently that farming entered the picture and that humans became exposed to cereals such as wheat and rye. As yet, our DNA has not had time to change to accommodate this change in diet. Until this change happens, cereals will top the list of food allergies.

What are the effects of a high-protein diet?

There are many people who claim that too much protein in the diet is harmful. However, this simply does not fit the facts. Scientific evidence suggests that those who live longest on the planet have the highest level of protein, especially animal protein, in the diet. Russians from the Caucasus Mountains, who are famous in Europe for their health and longevity, eat a diet with lots of meat and dairy produce. This is just one example of many. The claim that animal products shorten one's lifespan is not true. A high-protein diet is essential for good health.

A diet that is completely devoid of animal produce and which is based purely on plant produce is problematic. A vegetarian diet often lacks sufficient vitamin D (and other fat-soluble vitamins), leading to poor absorption of minerals such as calcium. Also, phytates in grains block the uptake of a number of minerals in the gut, which is why it's essential to pre-digest cereals (i.e. cereals have to be fermented or soaked in water before being used in cooking). In the modern world, this often doesn't happen.

One common deficiency in animals fed on grains is zinc deficiency. This can often lead to physical deformities. Zinc deficiency is not uncommon in humans and can result in learning difficulties, mental retardation, delayed sexual maturation, slow growth and many other problems. Up to one-third of the world's population is at risk of zinc deficiency; that's how important a public health issue it is. It's also the fifth leading risk factor for disease in the developing world.

Simply put, the ideal form of protein in the diet is animal protein, as this form of protein is complete and is easier for the gut to digest. I grew up listening to my family speak about the importance of protein and I learned about it at school and at university. In Africa, I saw the devastating effects of a lack of protein in young children, many of whom died as a result of having no protein in their diet. I now listen to a lot of nonsense being spoken about animal protein and animal fat. I can say without reservation that the basic foods needed every day in the diet are fat and protein in that order; fortunately, they occur together in Nature.

CARBOHYDRATE

Carbohydrate is described as the energy food or fuel for your body. It's true that carbohydrate does indeed provide a source of energy in the form of glucose. All living creatures, plants and animals alike, use glucose as a source of energy. However, glucose isn't the only source of energy. You may not know that fats are a much better source of energy in that they provide many more calories per gram. Carbohydrate includes starchy foods such as potatoes, rice, pasta and bread as well as sugary foods such as table sugar (sucrose), fruit sugar, such as fructose, and milk sugar, such as lactose.

Starchy foods such as potatoes are made up of long chains of glucose molecules. In the process of digestion, this long chain of glucose molecules gets broken down to individual glucose molecules, which can then be transported across the gut wall and into the bloodstream. It's dangerous to have too much glucose in the bloodstream, so the hormone insulin escorts it out of the bloodstream and into the cells of the body, where it's broken down to release energy. If the cell has sufficient supplies of stored energy, the glucose is stored for future use.

Although glucose is used in Nature to provide energy, we don't actually need to ingest it. The body has a very clever way of making glucose from fat in a process called gluconeogenesis (a nice simple term). This is because there was little starch available in the primitive diet, so the body needed other ways of getting a reliable supply of energy. Many people have existed, and some still do, without eating carbohydrate at all. Examples include the Masai, the Eskimo, the Inuit and Native Americans. Clearly, it is possible to survive without carbohydrate.

It is really only in the last century that the Western diet has included so much refined sugar. Prior to this, the only sugar consumed for the most part was honey or fruit sugar. Where sugar and starch are found in Nature, one also finds an array of vitamins and minerals, fibre, enzymes and also some fat and protein. Nature provides the enzymes to digest the carbohydrate as well as the essential vitamins and minerals to assist with absorption and metabolism. Nature also provides fibre to slow down the rate of absorption of glucose and to assist with bowel evacuation.

Refining carbohydrate strips the food of a lot of these extra vitamins, minerals, enzymes and fibre, making it harder for the body to digest and metabolise the food. It therefore means that your body's reserves of vitamins and minerals get called upon, thus depleting you of these essential elements. Because of the lack of fibre in refined carbohydrate, glucose levels in the bloodstream can rise sharply and ultimately predispose one to diabetes.

As I discussed in Chapter 2, the introduction of refined carbohydrate to isolated communities invariably led to a string of health problems appropriately called the diseases of civilisation: heart disease, diabetes, hypertension, obesity, arthritis, etc. Why is refined sugar in particular so damaging?

Table sugar (or sucrose, to give it its chemical name) is made up of two sugars: glucose and fructose. You're probably quite familiar with these two sugars already, as both are used in the home for baking and cooking. Glucose is relatively harmless, as it's Nature's energy-giving food and is used by every cell in every animal and plant. The real culprit is fructose, which in small quantities is fine, but in large quantities it wreaks havoc with the body's chemistry. Some describe it as a toxin or poison and I believe they are correct. It negatively affects the liver's ability to function in much the same way that alcohol does; in fact, many of the complications associated with alcohol toxicity mimic the complications associated with fructose toxicity.

All cells in the body can use glucose for energy or store it for future use. However, only the liver can use fructose, so the majority of the fructose absorbed heads straight for the liver, which is where all the damage is done. In small amounts, as in fruit, fructose causes no problems, but in high amounts it depletes the liver cells of energy, causes inflammation (hepatitis) and leads to the production of uric acid, which seems to be the key substance that causes a chain of additional health problems. What is interesting about the metabolism of fructose in the liver is the fact that most of it is converted to fat. This increase in the production of fat leads to an increase in bad cholesterol (LDL), which is implicated in heart disease (now you can see the link between sugar and heart disease). The increased production of fat also leads to increased fat in the liver (fatty liver) and other organs and the deposition of fat intra-abdominally (beer belly). Fructose does indeed appear to be the underlying cause of the obesity epidemic, as I have described in my e-book *The Big Fat Secret* (McKenna, 2012).

In the mid-1970s in the US, the food manufacturers decided to use a substance called high fructose corn syrup (HFCS) to replace fat, as it was very sweet and very cheap. Soon HFCS found its way into almost every processed food and drink. The food chemists knew the consequences of their actions, as the harmful effects of high levels of fructose were well documented in the 1950s and 60s and were highlighted in many of Professor John Yudkin's books (he was a professor of physiology in London who did a lot of research on fructose). However, they went ahead and did it anyhow. They have effectively destroyed the health of almost every nation on the planet who eat and drink processed foodstuffs. It's clear that these companies will do anything, including blatantly harming you and your family, for the sake of massive profits. This is the danger of allowing your society to be governed by money and by greed. We have seen the damage the banks have done; in the months and years to come, you will see the damage food companies have done.

The truth is that carbohydrate is not essential unless you're doing a lot of physical work or are a professional athlete. If you do eat carbohydrate, eat only wholemeal foods, such as wholewheat bread. However, all whole grains contain phytic acid, which blocks the absorption of certain minerals such as calcium, magnesium, zinc and copper. They are also hard to digest because of enzyme inhibitors that interfere with the action of digestive enzymes in the gut. This is why in Africa they always either soak or ferment grains before using them. So if you like to eat porridge oats, soak them overnight, as this will make them easier to digest. Many people who are allergic to cereals such as wheat may find that they can tolerate the cereal if it is pre-digested by soaking or fermenting it. Avoid sugar and all foods containing it and avoid any food containing high fructose corn syrup, which is labelled as corn syrup, fructose syrup or glucose-fructose. As you have learned above, sugar in large amounts is toxic.

To summarise so far, after water and good bacteria, fats are the next most important food group, followed by protein. Carbohydrate is the least important food group and the least important macronutrient. It is less important than the micronutrients minerals and vitamins, which I'll discuss next.

MINERALS

In my opinion, minerals are the most interesting and exciting part of our diet. They illustrate the link between us and the planet we inhabit. They also reflect our true origins as stellar beings. They are more important than vitamins by far. Allow me to explain what I mean.

Plants make food to feed the rest of creation. They do this by absorbing carbon dioxide (CO_2) from the air and water (H_2O) from the soil to make food in the form of glucose (which contains carbon, hydrogen and oxygen atoms). Plants also make protein, which contains nitrogen. Despite the fact that air has lots of nitrogen, plants are not able to use atmospheric nitrogen and so depend on a supply of nitrogen from the soil. But they cannot use inorganic nitrogen from soil, so they form a partnership with certain bacteria called nitrogen-fixing bacteria, which convert the nitrogen in soil into a form that plants can use, called organic nitrogen. In return the plant supplies the bacteria with food. Good trade! In this way, plants are able to make protein.

Plants also absorb many minerals from soil. These minerals get passed to you directly when you eat the plant raw or indirectly via animals that eat the plants. The mineral content of the soil is the single most important aspect of any discussion about human nutrition. If the soil is deficient, then your body will be deficient. We are directly and indirectly connected to the soil our food is grown in. The mineral content of the soil is the most important question to ask in any discussion about our food. Testing a soil for its mineral content is vitally important. If you grow your own vegetables, fruits or crops, get your soil tested regularly. If it's found to be deficient in one or more minerals, then correct the deficiency in the soil by adding a dressing of minerals and take a multi-mineral supplement yourself.

Minerals not only connect you to the very earth you stand on, but also to the universe. In particular, they connect you to dying stars, as this is where all minerals (calcium, magnesium, phosphorus, zinc, iron, etc.) are made. Hydrogen is the simplest atom. In stars like our sun, hydrogen atoms fuse together to form helium. To make more complicated atoms you need much higher temperatures, which only exist when a star is dying. It is only then that atoms such as carbon, oxygen and nitrogen (the basis of all food) can be formed and that life can become possible. It is only with even higher temperatures that other, bigger atoms can be formed, such as iron, zinc, calcium, etc. Dying stars are the origin of all food and all minerals that we know about. As the star dies it explodes and scatters these atoms across the universe, allowing life to occur and you and I to exist. You can see now why I say that minerals are bits of stardust and connect us to our origins. You are beginning to appreciate the true importance of minerals in the food chain. Without them, nothing else would exist. They are truly bits of magic.

We need seven minerals in large amounts – calcium, magnesium, phosphorus, potassium, sodium, chloride and sulphur – and many in trace amounts, too many to list. The exact number of trace minerals essential for life probably equates to the number of minerals found in the earth's crust, which is quite a lot. The exact role of many of these trace minerals is not known. In other words, we have much to learn.

We get most minerals and trace minerals from water, raw food or lightly cooked food and sea salt. What I find fascinating is the addition of soil to food and water in order to get enough minerals by many of the African tribes I have visited. In Europe, many people use clay for this purpose, such as the addition of bentonite clay to food by the French and by Alpine nations such as the Germans, Swiss, Austrians and Italians. Most of the minerals we need are found in food. These minerals play vital roles in many of the chemical reactions that take place in our cells. For example, iron is a positively charged mineral that binds to negatively charged sites on the haemoglobin molecule in red blood cells. In the act of binding, the iron changes the shape of the haemoglobin molecule, opening up a space for oxygen to now bind to haemoglobin. Without iron it would not be possible for oxygen to be transported around the body in the red blood cells. This oxygen is critical for cells to be able to convert food to energy.

Without iron made in a distant star in the galaxy, you would not exist, as you would not be able to get the benefit of the food you eat. All the minerals play equally important roles, which is why doctors measure many of these minerals when they do routine blood tests. Even though some minerals are only needed in tiny amounts, they are still essential for your survival. Interestingly, the body knows that too much of any of these minerals can be toxic, so the gut only absorbs what it needs at that time. In other words, we need a steady supply of minerals in our food on a daily basis to top up, so to speak.

There are a number of reasons why you may become deficient in minerals. Maybe the soil your vegetables were grown in is deficient, maybe the grass the cow ate was deficient, maybe your gut isn't functioning correctly or maybe other foods in your diet are blocking the absorption of these minerals.

As soil analyses have proven and tests done on fruits and vegetables have shown, the soil in market garden areas around many cities are depleted of minerals. Avoid supermarket vegetables and fruits and seek out a local farmer; better still, grow your own produce. Many people are now opting for the latter, as there has been a huge surge in the 'grow your own' movement. Alternatively, make sure you and your loved ones take a daily multi-mineral supplement, especially if you eat Western processed foods. Doctors who suggest that supplements aren't necessary because you will get all the micronutrients you need from your diet have simply never tested their patients for mineral deficiencies and don't understand nutrition, which isn't surprising since nutrition isn't taught at medical school. In my experience of living in the Western world, it's important to take vitamin and mineral supplements.

My favourite mineral is zinc. Let's take a closer look at it as a good example of how minerals operate in the body.

Zinc

A zinc deficiency can produce white spots on your nails and is one of the most common micronutrient deficiencies. Even mild zinc deficiency can have enormous consequences for a person's health. This is due to the fact that this trace mineral is required as a co-factor by over 200 enzyme reactions in various organs in the body, so a zinc deficiency can have widespread effects on your health. Signs of a deficiency include growth retardation, poor appetite, mental lethargy and increased susceptibility to infections. If your child has a poor appetite or has recurrent infections, a zinc supplement may be needed.

Zinc is now firmly established as a major protector of the immune system and an important weapon to fight disease. It has been clearly established that zinc is essential for immune system function carried out by white blood cells. *Acrodermatitis enteropathica* is a rare disorder that causes its victims to be more susceptible to infections and die young. These patients have defects in the activity of their white blood cells as well as in other parts of their immune system. The condition is reversible by the inclusion of zinc in the diet. Research on zinc deficiency has shown that there may be a decrease in circulating T-lymphocytes, which form another part of immunity, in people over the age of 70. This age group is one of the sections of the general population most at risk of recurrent infection. It has been suggested that the immune system may become weaker with age due to a fall in the zinc level at this stage of life. Other studies have shown that patients with AIDS have significantly lower blood levels of zinc when compared with a control group. This suggests a role for zinc supplementation in the elderly and in AIDS patients. The recommended daily allowance (RDA) for zinc is 15 mg a day for adults and 10 mg for children. I recommend a higher daily intake, as I have lived in southern Africa, where the soil is deficient in zinc, and have seen the effects of low zinc on the body. All the sports athletes in that part of the world are told to take zinc supplements (and magnesium as well). I also recommend a higher intake in order to quickly break a cycle of recurrent infections.

You can also supplement your daily intake of zinc by adding certain foods to your diet. The best dietary sources of zinc are whole grains, legumes and animal meats. Oysters have the highest levels of zinc. I normally recommend zinc supplementation initially for a three-month period and then assess after that if it is necessary to continue.

Certain foods can affect the way that your body is able to absorb and use zinc. Fibre, iron and calcium diminish the amount of zinc that you can absorb. Excessively high amounts of fibre can restrict the absorption of zinc quite significantly. Phytates in cereals can also bind to zinc and reduce its absorption.

There are no adverse effects associated with low-dose zinc supplementation. However, large doses of zinc – over 150 mg a day – may have a negative effect on your immunity. For this reason, correct dosage is important. In one particular study (Chandra, 1984), 11 men took 150 mg of zinc twice a day for six weeks. This resulted in a significant reduction in their immune systems. I recommend that you don't exceed 50 mg a day.

Because zinc competes with copper for absorption across the gut wall, high doses of zinc could create a copper deficiency. That's why some practitioners recommend including a small amount of copper when taking high doses of zinc. A dose of copper that is one-tenth of the zinc dosage is sufficient. In other words, if you're taking 50 mg of zinc, it may be advisable to take 5 mg of copper as well. Minerals are best taken as a multi-mineral. Rather than use individual micronutrients, it's best to take a broad spectrum supplement that includes all the minerals.

CLAY

As mentioned above, it's common practice in many parts of Africa and some parts of Europe to add clay to food or water. Certain clays are used in this way in health spas in the Alps. A teaspoon of clay is added to a glass of water and left to stand overnight. Upon waking, stir the water and drink it. Various types of clays are used, but bentonite is the one I'm most familiar with. It provides the body with an array of minerals. Clay also contains silicon, which can bind toxic metals and remove them from the body. Clay particles have a very large surface area relative to their size, allowing them to mop up toxic stuff. These clay particles have a negative charge and so attract positively charged particles such as metals. Beauty therapists use clays on the skin to remove toxins, but it can also be used internally, as is done in the spas of Europe.

VITAMINS

Many people regard vitamins and minerals as somewhat similar. There are some key differences between vitamins and minerals. Firstly, vitamins are complex molecules composed of carbon, hydrogen, oxygen and nitrogen, whereas minerals are very simple, usually existing as a charged atom (ion) or as a salt. Secondly, vitamins are easily damaged by factors such as temperature, pressure and radiation; minerals are not damaged by these factors. Therefore, freshness is important in terms of vitamin content but unimportant regarding mineral content. If a mineral is present in a food, it will remain until the food is eaten. However, cooking methods can alter the vitamin content significantly. For example, vitamin C is largely destroyed by cooking. Thus, minerals are simple, basic structures, whereas vitamins are chemically much more complex. It is this complexity that makes them more susceptible to damage. All minerals must be obtained from food, whereas some vitamins, such as vitamin D, can be manufactured by the body.

Vitamins are even more complex in that many of them need additional co-factors to operate effectively. For example, vitamin C needs certain minerals, rutin, bioflavonoids and other substances to function. Vitamins often do not exist as single entities but as a group of complex molecules, many of which have yet to be discovered. Vitamin B complex has at least 17 components that we know of, which appear to work together synergistically. Vitamin D has 12 components and vitamin P at least five. Because of their complex nature and the many constituents, vitamins are very difficult to manufacture in pill form, making food the best source of obtaining them.

For the most part, vitamins seem to work as antioxidants

that protect the cells from damage or they work as facilitators of enzyme reactions, i.e. they work as co-factors helping certain chemical reactions take place. Vitamin C is an antioxidant while vitamin B1 is a co-factor.

The food processing industry may add vitamins at low levels for advertising purposes but then proceed to damage these vitamins by subjecting them to high heat and pressure. In addition, sugar added to the food will deplete the body of some of the B vitamins. Long periods of high heat used in canning foods can also destroy certain vitamins. Interestingly, sun drying can actually enhance vitamin content, e.g. in sun-dried fruits. The traditional methods of treating foods were much wiser and safer.

One vitamin in particular is worthy of mention. Vitamin A is the reason why I got interested in nutrition. I remember reading an article on the positive benefits of vitamin A supple-mentation in reducing infections in children born to mothers who were HIV positive. It was a study carried out in Durban, South Africa, in the early 1990s. It made me acutely aware why HIV infection is so prevalent in southern Africa: it all came down to poor nutrition.

Because I have always had a strong interest in digestive problems, vitamin A was of interest to me, as it assists in the digestion of protein in the stomach by stimulating the secretion of digestive juices. However, it does a lot more than this. According to Dr Weston Price the body can't utilise protein, minerals or water-soluble vitamins (C and B complex) without sufficient vitamin A. Hence, vitamin A could be regarded as the single most important vitamin and possibly micronutrient. Animal sources of vitamin A (eggs, liver, cod liver oil, seafood, milk, butter) are much easier for the body to use; vegetable sources (any green, yellow or orange vegetable, such as carrots, spinach or cabbage) are harder for the body to use, as the vegetable form of vitamin A, beta carotene, needs to be converted in the body to retinol, which is the form the body needs. Animal sources of vitamin A do not need to be converted, as they are supplied in the form of retinol. The conversion of beta carotene to retinol can be difficult for some people, especially infants and young children, diabetics and for those with an underactive thyroid (hypothyroidism). According to Dr Price's findings and to many other researchers since then, the healthiest people on the planet have the highest intake of vitamin A.

Vitamin A is probably the most powerful antioxidant of all. It has been researched extensively for its ability to prevent cancer, even in those at greater risk than the average person. The increase in incidence of certain types of cancer has been linked by some researchers to low vitamin A levels (Boik, 2001). The results of these studies show that lung cancer in particular is associated with low levels of vitamin A in the diet as well as cancers of the larynx, mouth, oesophagus, stomach, colon, prostate and cervix (Boik, 2001). Research from Japan (Tsubono, 1999) has shown that those who consume foods rich in vitamin A are less likely to develop a whole range of cancers. Research from the Philippines (De Luca, 1995) has shown that the administration of vitamin A has the ability to reduce cellular abnormalities pre-cancer state, especially in the mouth and in the cervix.

Vitamin A deficiency is one of the most serious nutritional deficiencies across the globe. Severe vitamin A deficiency occurs commonly in the developing world and I have personally seen many children in Africa with it. Interestingly, I have also seen evidence of it here in Europe amongst people with malabsorption and in people using slimming pills, which block the absorption of fat in the gut, causing fatty stools. Signs of deficiency include:

- Dry eyes
- Difficulty seeing well in dim light (night blindness)
- Dry skin
- Recurrent infections
- In children in Africa, poor growth and development (failure to thrive).

Many people know that vitamin A is important for vision and for the skin (beauty therapists use it to treat damaged skin and to rejuvenate skin). What is less well known is its ability to protect against infections. A clinical trial carried out in Papua New Guinea in the late 1990s (Shankar, 1999) showed the protective effect of vitamin A supplements when children contracted malaria. Vitamin A was able to significantly reduce the parasite load, thereby preventing serious complications, including death. Malaria is the biggest killer worldwide and is estimated to have killed half of all humans who have ever lived.

Vitamin A is one of the fat-soluble vitamins. It's stored in the body, so it's possible to overdose on it. The recommended intake of retinol for adults is approximately 1,000 mg a day. Pregnant women and breastfeeding mothers require a little bit more – up to 1,200 mg a day. It's possible to use higher doses, but remember that it's stored in the body and so can be toxic at very high doses. It's best to eat lots of foods rich in vitamin A, which is what Nature intended, rather than take pills.

ENZYMES

If I had written this book 20 years ago I probably would not have included a section on enzymes. The study of enzymes and the role they play in Nature is relatively new in the field of nutrition. Today we have identified thousands of enzymes, which seem to play a role in just about every chemical reaction that happens in the body. They basically speed up chemical reactions by bringing all the components together to allow reactions to happen.

To help bring the components up close and personal, so to speak, enzymes employ minerals and vitamins. When a vitamin or mineral attaches to an enzyme to help it speed up a chemical reaction, the vitamin or mineral is referred to as a co-factor. This is a principal role of vitamins and minerals. For example, zinc is known to be a co-factor in over 200 enzyme reactions in various parts of the body. When glucose enters the cell it's broken down in a series of enzyme reactions to carbon dioxide and water. Magnesium and the B vitamins play roles as co-factors in some of these reactions. Enzymes could be regarded as facilitators of chemical reactions and they employ the help of micronutrients as co-workers.

You're probably quite familiar with the digestive enzymes in your digestive tract that break down your food to facilitate absorption across the gut wall. This is one class of enzyme, but there are two other classes as well: metabolic enzymes, which facilitate all the chemical reactions in the cells of the body; and the third class, called food enzymes, which is what I wish to discuss now.

Raw foods sometimes contain enzymes that help the process of digestion. The food is giving you a present of digestive enzymes to ease the burden on your pancreas. It's making the job of converting the food into a bio-available form that much easier. Hence, raw foods become an important part of any diet. We tend to eat raw fruits and sometimes vegetables in salads and some people drink raw milk, but primitive peoples often eat some of their meat raw and on occasion raw fish as well. What they do not eat raw or cooked, they will ferment over a period of time, which can enhance the nutritional value of the food. Fermented dairy products such as soured milk are not only rich in bacteria, but rich in enzymes as well. For this reason, it's important to consume fermented products such as fermented vegetables (sauerkraut) or fermented soya beans (tofu and miso).

Grains, nuts and seeds are rich in enzymes but also contain enzyme inhibitors that make them a bit hard on the digestive tract. To get rid of these enzyme inhibitors, certain techniques have been used over the centuries, such as sprouting, soaking food in water with a little lemon juice added, fermenting or sourdough leavening. Most fruit and vegetables have little in the way of enzymes, with a few notable exceptions. Pineapple and pawpaw (papaya) are rich in enzymes and are used by some companies that manufacture digestive enzymes for sale in health shops. Many tropical fruits, such as kiwi, avocado, mango, dates, banana and plantain, also contain enzymes.

High heat destroys all the natural enzymes in food. The process of pasteurisation kills bad bacteria by the use of high heat; effectively, by boiling the milk. This not only destroys all the bacteria but all the enzymes as well, making the milk much harder to digest. The activity of one particular enzyme, alkaline phosphatase, is measured after heating the milk. If it's zero, then the milk can be deemed pasteurised. Now you understand all the political fuss about trying to keep raw milk available for people. Politicians are trying to ban the sale of raw milk and others who use raw milk are opposing them. I'm in agreement that raw milk should be made available to people. Milk has become too commercial a product and there is too much interference in the production of milk and too many middlemen, especially the supermarkets. I'm strongly in favour of connecting consumers with farmers and cutting out all the food manufacturers and supermarkets. I do like raw milk, but I don't eat a high raw food diet.

Personally, I'm not a great fan of a raw food diet. Culturally I was brought up on mostly cooked food and I have continued this pattern of eating. However, mentally I understand the need for a lot of raw or fermented food in the diet, but emotionally I haven't succumbed to the idea. I do eat salads (occasionally) and I do eat lots of fruit and try to get raw milk, but I'm afraid to say the rest of my diet is cooked. For me, Ireland is too cold to survive on mostly raw or fermented food. I hear others speak about nutrition and saying that 80 per cent of your diet should be raw food. Good for them if they can do it, but I enjoy what I eat and have evolved a way of eating that's good for me. I'm tuned in to my body well enough to know what it needs.

SALT

We humans evolved from the sea and the composition of our bodies reflects this. I said earlier in this chapter that we are mostly water. That water is mostly saltwater. The water in our bloodstream and in tissue fluid has sodium chloride dissolved in it. Both sodium and chloride are important for health.

Salt sold in supermarkets, like much of the food sold there, is highly refined. Even a lot of sea salt is refined as well. It undergoes chemical changes in the refining process that removes most of the magnesium and other minerals. The best salt is sun-dried sea salt, which is not refined and so is rich in sodium chloride and in many other minerals as well. It's best to buy salt in a health food shop and ask for unrefined, sun-dried sea salt.

———

In summary, the main constituents of a healthy diet are water, good bacteria, fats, protein, minerals and vitamins with a minimum amount of carbohydrate, unless you're expending a lot of energy at work. Part of the diet should be raw food. Having said all of that, I'm now going to examine some of the controversies surrounding some of these foods.

The human body is very simple in one sense and highly complex in another sense. It needs basic, simple, natural foods such as those listed above to function effectively. However, the way these foods combine in the body is truly magical and complex. We need to trust in Nature and in the foods she provides us with.

We have been deliberately led away from this simple, natural diet in favour of denatured food. We have been deliberately misled about cholesterol, about sugar and even about animal protein. If you confuse people enough, you can control them.

We have been poisoned with high fructose corn syrup, which is causing health problems of a magnitude this world has never seen. Later in this book I'll mention some of the artificial sweeteners, such as aspartame, which is being blamed for the sudden rise in brain tumours since its introduction in 1981. We have been deliberately misinformed by governments, by the WHO, by the medical profession, by dieticians and by many other organisations and professional bodies. Why? For profit via control of the food chain. You are being conned, big time.

Let's now look at the elements of a healthy diet again from a different perspective. Let's start with water.

WATER

I grew up drinking well water and later, tap water. At the age of 15 I went on a school trip to France and was surprised to see people drinking water from a plastic bottle. In my innocence, I believed that water was free, plentiful and safe to drink.

It's now almost impossible to find clean, safe water to drink. We have polluted the water table, streams and rivers with agricultural chemicals. Tap water is laden with chemicals and because of its high solid content, it's unhealthy to drink. That leaves bottled water, which is the best option even if it's in a plastic bottle. Alternatively, get a reverse osmosis filter to purify your tap water.

Spa mineral water from Belgium is an excellent mineral water available in the UK but not in Ireland. It has won many awards over the years. It has a very low TDS level and so has a high level of purity. It comes from an artesian well in the town of Spa in Belgium. Glacial water such as Isklar from Norway, artesian well water and volcanic water such as Volvic are also good, as they come from the belly of the earth or from melting glaciers. These are the purest forms of water.

There have been problems with bad bugs in the tap water supply in many countries. This leads to acute illness. What's a bit more serious is the presence of metals in the water supply. An article in the *Irish Examiner* in 2013 stated that an Environmental Protection Agency report showed that 42 local water supplies in Ireland had unacceptable levels of lead (O'Doherty, 2013). Lead is a highly toxic metal, which is why it was removed from petrol, paint and solder. It causes chronic ill health.

Chlorine is added to tap water. Chlorine not only kills bad bacteria, it also kills the good bacteria in your body. Fluoride is also added to tap water. Fluoride is an enzyme inhibitor that can cause bone loss and has now been implicated in the development of bone cancer. In 1990 the American National Toxicology Program reported a clear linkage between flouride and the malignant bone cancer osteosarcoma (Epstein, 1998). This cancer is on the increase, is almost invariably fatal and affects young children and adolescents (Epstein, 1998: 390). This is a good reason to ban the fluoridation of water.

Avoid tap water regardless of where you live and try to get the best bottled water you can. The rationale behind water purification plants operated by your local council is to remove as much debris as possible and to kill bugs. It has nothing at all to do with producing water as close to its natural state as possible; it has nothing to do with healthy water for the human body. The sole rationale is safety. Safe water is not healthy water. The two objectives are poles apart. Chlorine will make your water safe, but who wants to drink swimming pool water?

FATS

Animal fats have been demonised, as has cholesterol. It's as if these two foods were responsible for striking people down in the prime of their lives. Doctors advise their patients to cut down on eggs, butter and cheese and to eat lean meats. Everyone follows the same advice, as they wish to prevent heart attacks.

I'm sad to say that the advice is totally incorrect. What do I mean by this? Firstly, the terminology is all wrong. Cholesterol and animal fat are completely different substances with completely different functions in the body. Cholesterol is not a fat at all. Chemically, it bears no relation to fat.

Secondly, when we use the term 'bad cholesterol', there is no such thing, as all cholesterol is good and necessary. This kind of useless term demonises a food that is critical for human health. We should be using the term low-density lipoprotein (LDL). There's no need to add 'cholesterol' after LDL.

Thirdly, there is no hard scientific evidence to substantiate the idea that any type of fat is bad for you, including animal fat, and there's definitely no evidence that animal fat causes heart disease. The Framingham Heart Study – the most famous medical study ever done on heart disease – has shown there is no link with animal fat. So why persist with this nonsense? You're being misled, misinformed and wrongly advised.

As I've shown in my book *The Big Fat Secret* (McKenna, 2012), however, there is hard scientific evidence linking sugar intake with heart disease. This information is kept hidden from you by lies, deceit and misinformation. However, it will not remain hidden for much longer. The controversy about fat and cholesterol is really just a smoke screen to hide the truth. Use fat and cholesterol freely.

PROTEIN

There is much controversy surrounding the link between dairy products and cancer. The link between casein, a milk protein, and various forms of cancer has been known for some time but was highlighted in 2006 with the publication of *The China Study* (Campbell and Campbell, 2006). In this book, the research does indeed show a link between casein and certain cancers, notably liver cancer. On the basis of this research, it's possible to advise people to be cautious about commercial, pasteurised milk. However, there is no problem with the whey protein found in milk.

What I don't like about the book is its conclusion that not just dairy, but all animal protein should be avoided. The authors spend most of the book advocating a vegan diet rather than dealing with the evidence from their research in China. There are some fundamental errors in their conclusions. They ignore the many tribes of people in the world who have thrived on animal protein for centuries and who show no evidence of liver cancer or any other cancer. Some of these tribes, such as the Fulani and Masai in Africa, consume a lot of milk protein. They also ignore the fact that their source of casein was from pasteurised milk, not raw milk. Maybe it's the pasteurisation process that's altering the casein and making it cancer promoting.

Until this controversy about casein is settled, I would advise caution in the use of processed milk such as pasteurised milk and opt for raw milk. Avoid all commercial dairy products such as cheese, yoghurt and ice cream; cream and butter are composed of animal fat, so they should be okay to use. Better still, use goat's milk or sheep's milk as alternatives. Highly commercial products such as cow's milk are big business. Just because it's endorsed by your government or your health authority doesn't mean it's safe. My motto is: if there's the slightest risk of harm, avoid it completely.

FOOD ADDITIVES

You will learn quite soon via the national press about the damage that certain food additives are doing to our health. In particular, much research has focused on the artificial sweeteners aspartame, sucralose and acesulfame K. These sweeteners have been endorsed as safe, yet they have consistently been shown to be harmful to people and to experimental animals.

These sweeteners are added to a number of conventional drugs, such as Calpol, Calcichew and cold and flu remedies. They're also added to vitamin supplements, so it's best to buy all vitamins in a health shop. Sucralose has been shown to damage the bacterial flora of the gut and predispose people to colitis, Crohn's disease and bowel cancer. Aspartame has been shown to cause leukaemia in humans. So throw out the diet drinks and check all medicine for the addition of these additives.

They are so toxic to humans that I've written a special section on them in Chapter 7. Please read this section and clean out your cupboards if you wish to stay healthy and well. I would urge someone to develop an app for use on mobile phones that shows the presence of these additives to save the bother of reading labels. I know there's an app called Fooducate where you can scan the barcode of a food item and it will indicate the presence of genetically modified foods, but I'm not aware of any other apps for use on your mobile to do with food. Please feel free to write to me or e-mail me if you come across any of these apps.

In the next chapter I want to examine where farming has gone wrong and the consequences for us, the consumers.

Chapter 6
What Has Gone Wrong?

WHAT HAPPENED TO FARMING?

A meeting took place in a city in Germany in 1909 that was to change the face of farming many years later. This meeting was between senior chemists from BASF, the biggest chemical company in the world at that time, and a brilliant research chemist who worked in the Karlsruhe Technical University, Fritz Haber. Haber wanted to demonstrate a chemical experiment that was truly revolutionary. He showed how he had devised a method of using nitrogen in the air to make ammonia, an organic form of nitrogen that plants could use.

This may not sound very revolutionary to you, but it had the potential to eliminate famine, which was the scourge of mankind. It had the potential to double crop yields and to feed the ever-growing population in Europe in particular. It would also mean massive profits for the chemical company that utilised the technique to make lots of nitrogen fertiliser.

Prior to this landmark discovery, we were dependent on a supply of guano from Peru or sodium nitrate from Chile, both far from Europe and expensive to transport, as a source of nitrogen to enhance plant growth. The possibility of making organic nitrogen in a factory in Europe could change all of that, and if it could be produced at low cost, there was also the potential to export it to other countries.

Plants can't utilise atmospheric nitrogen, as it's in an inorganic form and thus hard for the plant to absorb. Plants rely on bacteria in the soil to convert inorganic nitrogen to organic nitrogen, which is absorbed through the roots. Fritz Haber had discovered a way of doing what bacteria do: he discovered a means of chemically converting nitrogen into ammonia. This had never been done before and excited the visiting chemists from BASF that afternoon in 1909.

BASF decided to see if the chemistry experiment could be used to make large quantities of ammonia on an industrial scale. Five years later, in 1914, BASF was producing four tons of ammonia a day; by 1918, they were producing nearly 300 tons a day in a specially built factory in Saxony. Without ammonia, Germany's Second Reich war effort would have failed, as ammonia was also used to make munitions. Fritz Haber won the Nobel Prize for Chemistry after the war for his synthesis of ammonia.

After the war, Imperial Chemical Industries (ICI) was formed in Britain. Since they had learned the secrets of how to make ammonia from the Germans, they began to produce it on an industrial scale for use across the British empire. The idea of using artificial fertiliser on their soil didn't sit well with farmers, who were very sceptical. They were even more sceptical when they realised they would have to pay for it. To try to convince everyone of the benefits, ICI set up an experimental farm near Maidenhead, Berkshire, and employed a professor of botany, Professor Keeble, to take charge.

Professor Keeble's experiments did indeed show a much higher crop yield with ammonia fertiliser. However, there was now a recession in Britain and farmers weren't convinced about his experiments and weren't going to spend their hard-earned cash on something that bacteria in the soil could do already. Clover is a plant that has lots of these bacteria attached to the roots, so farmers depend on clover to supply the soil with lots of organic nitrogen. Farmers were adamant that their cash wasn't going to be spent on artificial chemicals. In the lead-up to the Second World War, ICI produced tons of stocks of ammonia fertiliser but couldn't sell it. Having failed with the farmers, ICI decided to try to influence the government instead.

They initially failed there too, but with the onset of the Second World War and the problem with imports of cereals being blocked by the Germans, the UK had to become self-reliant and food production became a major issue. The Ministry of Agriculture and the Ministry of Food were now in control of food production and realised that if Britain was to survive, everything possible had to be done to increase the quantity of food grown. ICI's experiments helped convince the government that nitrogen fertiliser was the way to go. Because politicians, not farmers, were in control of agriculture, ICI found a use for their stocks of fertiliser and so all farmers were forced to use it, whether they liked it or not. After the war, the government introduced guaranteed prices for farm produce, which meant the farmer got paid irrespective of the quality of the produce. This was where farming got corrupted. Suddenly, quantity became more important than quality; in other words, the more you produced, the more you got paid, irrespective of quality.

The second mistake the government made was to introduce special subsidies on fertilisers. The idea was to help farmers produce higher yields, but in effect this allowed the chemical industry to gain a foothold on food production. One of the problems with getting a higher yield from a field is that you put greater demands on the soil. Eventually it became apparent that crops grown with artificial fertilisers were a lot weaker and more prone to fungal infections. The cell walls of the cereal were weaker and the plants were less resistant to insects and fungi. The crops were literally being forced out of the ground, regardless of quality. The farmers were won over because they were getting paid, ICI was happy, as they were making millions, and the consumer got lots of food.

To help solve the problems with insects and fungi, ICI developed chemicals to kill these pests, and again the government assisted by making subsidies available for farmers to purchase these. Yet again there was co-operation between industry and the government to control food production. Traditional methods of farming were discouraged and the new chemical methods were introduced wholesale across the country. The ecology of the soil was destroyed, rivers and lakes were polluted and worse still, the water table, which was a source of drinking water for many, was contaminated. Even the food produced from these crops is routinely contaminated with chemicals. What is a real tragedy is that we now have a generation of young farmers who believe it's nearly impossible to grow crops without artificial fertilisers and chemical sprays. Because of political decisions made during and after the war, chemical farming has effectively replaced traditional farming. We now call the latter organic farming, which is really just chemical-free farming.

There's another side to this story that's worth mentioning. To gain even greater control of agriculture, in the 1960s and

70s the chemical companies bought seed companies and developed varieties of rice and wheat that yield more protein but require more chemicals to grow. These crops do produce more protein but are deficient in minerals and antioxidants and so do not supply your body with the nutrients that Nature intended. This renders people more susceptible to disease. Worse still, the chemicals used on these cereals end up in the food you eat, making you sick. Effectively, we have chemical companies controlling the genetics of seed production and controlling how the crops that feed you are grown. This is bad news for everyone concerned, but particularly for consumers.

Nitrogen fertilisers have had the biggest impact on farming and on the environment. They have led to the destruction of the structure of the soil. Nitrogen fertilisers have altered the aeration and drainage of soil. In other words, they alter the air pockets in the soil and the water content of the soil. Since air and water are important for the survival of soil organisms such as microbes, the whole microbial content of the soil changes. This can deplete the soil of important minerals.

Nitrogen fertilisers also damage lakes and rivers in that they promote the growth of algae, which uses up all the oxygen and so kills off fish and other organisms in the river or lake. This has had catastrophic effects on our environment. Nitrogen in our water table, which supplies many wells with drinking water, causes a range of health problems. Too much nitrogen in the body is toxic. It's particularly dangerous for pregnant women, as it's known to cause miscarriages, birth defects and thyroid disorders. In infants it can cause blue baby syndrome because it interferes with the ability of red blood cells to carry oxygen to the tissues of the body. However, the real worry about nitrates is their ability to form carcinogenic compounds in the body, which have been linked with cancer in almost every organ in a range of experimental animals.

But that's not the only damaging consequence of modern farming methods. The farmer also uses a range of chemicals to grow the cereal that ends up on your table as bread or breakfast cereal. Weed killers such as isoproturon and pendimethalin are sprayed on in the autumn. Insecticides such as lambda-cyhalothrin are used at the same time. Fungicides such as Propiconazole are used in spring along with a mixture of growth hormones such as chlormequat. As the plants grow taller and thus weaker in resistance, they are subjected to another dose of fungicides and growth hormones. Then, during the stage of rapid plant growth, another dose of the same chemicals is sprayed on again. When the flag leaf (top leaf) appears, guess what – it gets yet another dose of fungicide.

This incessant need to keep spraying the plants indicates there is clearly something weakening the plant in the first place: the use of nitrogen fertilisers. Now you see the devastating effect Fritz Haber's invention has had, even if he did win a Nobel Prize for it.

Do these chemicals end up in your food? Tests are carried out in most countries to establish the presence of chemical residues in food. Chemical residues of weed killers, insecticides and hormones routinely show up in breads and in breakfast cereals. In Europe the three most common were chlormequat, a growth hormone; glyphosate, a weed killer (more commonly known as Roundup); and malathion, an insecticide. The levels found were worryingly high.

As with the issue of fructose in the diet and with other

chemicals such as artificial sweeteners, it's not the acute dosage that is of concern, but rather the chronic dosage over years of exposure. Strange as it may seem, no long-term studies have been done on exposure to the chemicals used by farmers on crops that you consume. That is a public disgrace. If these chemicals are found in your food, you need to know the consequences of long-term exposure. It is high time public money was used to investigate this topic fully.

A group of Canadian doctors was so concerned about people being exposed to a cocktail of chemicals day after day, year after year that they decided to review a lot of the research done to date. The Ontario College of Family Physicians study, published in April 2012, found definite links between pesticide exposure and various health problems, such as damage to the central nervous system (brain and spinal cord) and respiratory problems as well as a whole range of fertility and reproductive issues in both sexes. This isn't surprising, given that malathion is a dangerous chemical and is known to cause serious health problems, including cancer. Roundup, or glyphosate, is known to damage the central nervous system as well as causing respiratory difficulties such as asthma and bronchitis. What this study clearly indicates is the serious risks to pregnant women and young children. This study shows that pesticide exposure during pregnancy, especially the first trimester, can result in low birth weight, asthma, low IQ, learning problems, ADHD and autism as well as anti-social behaviour in older children.

Various studies (Ontario College of Family Physicians, 2012) found significant levels of pesticides in the breast milk and umbilical cord of mothers after birth, indicating previous exposure. These studies call for a radical reduction in the exposure of pregnant women and young children to pesticides in the environment and in foods grown using chemical sprays. I would call for a ban on the use of all chemicals used in the food chain. They are not necessary and are a consequence of using nitrogen fertilisers. By going back to the old ways of growing crops, we will safeguard the health of all, but we will have to endure lower yields.

There is a much more sinister side to modern farming methods. It involves the use of genetically modified (GM) seeds by one company in particular, Monsanto, the chemical company that also makes Roundup. They supply farmers with corn and soy seeds to grow crops. Nothing really new in that, but what's particularly sinister about this is that all research on these GM seeds must be approved by Monsanto. In other words, if I'm a scientist or doctor wishing to perform experiments using GM seeds, I have to apply to Monsanto for a supply of seeds and my research can't be published without Monsanto's approval. In other words, Monsanto can effect-ively block all adverse reports on their GM seeds, thereby making it impossible for researchers to alert the rest of us to potential problems. This is the present legal position. You might ask how this was allowed in the 'free' world. This is a worrying development in the control that chemical com-panies have been allowed to exert on food production.

It's time for us all to call for an independent inquiry into the links between certain food manufacturers and chemical companies such as Monsanto and the US and UK governments. Enough is enough. For example, there appears to be a revolving door between Monsanto and the US government. Many

Monsanto employees go on to work for the US Administration, e.g. Donald Rumsfeld. They end up as part of the government or as advisors to the government. Monsanto and the US government are morphing into one. Conflict of interest isn't a concept that bothers these people. Promoting vested interests in the US and passing laws to protect these vested interests is perfectly acceptable. How corrupt does Western society have to become before we all wake up and rebel?

It's time for a new way of doing things. This is one of the reasons I have said that the most important political act you perform each day is what food you buy and where you buy it. Think long and hard about the food you buy. You and only you have the power to make this a better world for our children. If you continue to buy processed foods, you are essentially making yourself dependent on the food companies and chemical companies that have no qualms about poisoning you. Yes, they are poisoning you, and worse still, they are getting away with it.

Also, as a taxpayer you are funding, via government subsidies, these chemical companies and allowing them to produce not just low-quality food, but toxic food. By your silence and inertia, you are effectively agreeing to this wasteful and harmful method of farming. We all have endorsed low-quality food for the sake of higher yields and endorsed the steady degradation of our planet via fertilisers and chemical sprays. We can change it all by taking a bit more time shopping for healthier foods. More on this later.

In summary, farming has undergone an amazing revolution since the Second World War. It has moved away from traditional values and wisdom to becoming dependent on harmful chemicals. Farming has lost its way and has become reflective of society as a whole, where money has become the god. Farming has become about producing more and more instead of about producing the healthiest food possible.

WHAT HAPPENED TO FOOD?

Having examined what has happened in the farmer's world, I'm now going to examine what happened to the food after it left the farmer's gate. I'm not going to discuss all food and all methods of production. Instead, I'm going to use milk as an example. Milk is an interesting product to look at to get a view of what has happened over the past 50 years. It illustrates very well how science, politics, industry and economics have been used to pull the wool over our eyes.

When I was growing up, raw, unpasteurised milk was the norm in the country, even though pasteurised milk was available by then. Then in the 1950s, there was a suggestion (also called a theory) that saturated or animal fat may be linked with the increase in heart disease. Because of some badly conducted research in the US, people were advised to reduce the level of animal fat in the diet. This then led to the multi-million-dollar industry manufacturing margarine spreads, low-fat milk, low-fat cheese, etc. to supposedly protect us all from coronary artery disease (blocked arteries). The theory was that animal fat blocked arteries and so led to heart disease. By the late 1970s it became apparent that this theory was incorrect, yet no public advice was given to advise people of this. Until today, the general public have been no wiser. Doctors are afraid to tell you, as a lot of funding for research comes from the food industry. Dieticians are also afraid to tell you, as they are also funded by the food industry. The health authorities won't inform you either, nor will politicians, as they are frightened of the severe criticism that would follow and would expose the true relationship between food companies and government. The truth never sees the light of day and confusion reigns.

Far from being harmful, animal fats play the single most important role in human nutrition. They are the building blocks of every cell in your body. They provide essential vitamins and are one of the best anti-cancer substances in the food chain. Animal fats are extremely important during pregnancy and for growing children. To demonise animal fat is to demonise Nature.

The other important food group is protein. In Nature, protein is always found in combination with fats or oils. Milk is the perfect example of this combination. Milk is often called the perfect food – that is, until the low-fat idea emerged. Milk has effectively been undermined by the very structures in our society that we rely on for impartial advice: the medical profession, dieticians, the health authorities and the government.

Today we are finding that more and more people are developing an allergy to or an intolerance of milk. This has happened gradually over the past 50 years and is now reaching epidemic levels. I have seen this in my own practice over the past 25 years. Milk's composition has been altered so much that what used to be a healthy food has now become a source of illness for more and more people. Doctors used to recommend raw milk as a cure for a host of complaints. In 1929, Dr Crewe of the famous Mayo Foundation wrote that raw milk can be used to improve heart disease, diabetes, obesity and tuberculosis.

Science is now proving him to be correct. Raw milk straight from the animal is now proving to be not just an excellent source of nutrition, but a powerful medicine. Modern pasteurised milk is proving to be the exact opposite.

Let's go back to basics for a moment. Grass is a highly fibrous material and impossible for humans to digest. On the other hand, cows have a rumen in which fibrous grasses are broken down and converted to food due to the presence of lots of microbes in the rumen. Cows can therefore convert grass into milk. The quality of the grass determines the quality of the milk. Poor-quality grass leads to poor-quality milk and as a consequence, poor health of the person drinking the milk. Good-quality grass produces good-quality milk and good health of the person drinking the milk. The fresher the grass, the better the milk will be; the best grass is the first grasses of spring. Milk from cows fed on fresh grass has high levels of the fat-soluble vitamins A, D, E and K as well as lots of good cholesterol and the fats so essential for good health. Milk from grass-fed cows also contains high levels of essential fatty acids (omega 3 fats), especially conjugated linoleic acid (CLA), which has been shown to have strong anti-cancer properties. Even small amounts of CLA can significantly reduce the risk of developing cancer. Organically produced milk is even richer in nutrients – it has been shown to have up to 50 per cent more vitamin E and up to 75 per cent more vitamin A as well as being up to 30 per cent higher in omega 3 fats. These levels are even higher in spring, when the cattle have greater access to natural green pastures.

So what's wrong with pasteurised milk? Firstly, the process of pasteurisation is designed to kill potentially harmful bugs such as bovine tuberculosis by subjecting the milk to high heat for a short time. High temperatures alter proteins in the milk, such as casein. It also alters the enzymes present in milk (raw milk is full of enzymes to help you digest it). Pasteurisation effectively destroys these enzymes, making it much more difficult to digest the milk and benefit from the nutrients contained in it.

Secondly, heating the milk destroys the beneficial bacteria present in raw milk. Heat not only destroys bad bacteria, but also all of the good ones that are essential for good health, such as *Lactobacillus acidophilus* and *Bifidobacterium bifidum*. All pasteurised milk products are deficient in good bacteria. If you want to know whether or not a milk has been pasteurized, let it stand at room temperature for a few days. If it sours or curds, then good bacteria are present and the milk has not been pasteurised. Soured milk has been very important in the history of every culture on this planet, with the exception of modern Westerners. It has played a key role in the diet of all of these cultures because it was used to replace good bacteria in the body on a daily basis. I grew up drinking buttermilk, the Fulani in West Africa use curded milk (what we would call yoghurt) and today we have 'live' yoghurt available in a few supermarkets. Most of the yoghurts sold in supermarkets are useless and potentially harmful, as they are made with pasteurised milk and have had sugar added. Try to get a yoghurt with living cultures in your local health shop or farm shop, or better still, get a yoghurt maker and make your own.

The third reason to avoid pasteurised milk is because of the addition of chemicals after heat treatment. These chemicals are added to suppress odour (boiled milk can smell). Other chemicals are added to improve taste. Synthetic vitamin D_2 or D_3 is then added. All in all, it's quite a chemically treated product.

The fourth reason to avoid pasteurised milk is because the milk may contain antibiotics. Despite the fact that mastitis is common in dairy herds and that milk should not be sent to the creamery while treating the mastitis with antibiotics, chemists have devised masking agents that conceal the presence of the antibiotic in the milk. After all, farmers would have to forfeit the income from milk sales if they withheld milk every time their cattle developed mastitis. The problem is that the antibiotics in milk can cause significant problems for the consumer. They can cause allergic reactions and gut problems such as cramps, flatulence, bloating and diarrhoea. The antibiotics can also encourage the development of antibiotic resistance.

The final reason to abstain from pasteurised milk is the fact that it may be homogenised. This is a process in which the fat globules in milk are forcibly broken down into smaller globules so that the fat is distributed throughout the milk rather than rising to the top. Homogenisation is carried out under high pressure and it generates high temperatures, effectively producing a second pasteurisation process. It's done purely to increase the shelf life of milk. Many researchers are linking homogenisation with the development of allergic reactions to milk (Oski, 1992). Other researchers have linked it with heart disease (Oster, 1971; Oster and Ross, 1973; Oster, Oster and Ross, 1974).

Commonly available milk in your local supermarket is best avoided. It simply does not resemble the raw milk I was raised on. If you want a good source of milk, log on to the internet and find a local farmer willing to supply you with raw milk. The hygiene standards for farms that sell milk directly to the public have to be much higher than farms that send their milk to the creamery. In this way, the public is protected.

WHAT HAS BEEN DONE TO THE COW?

There seems to be an insatiable desire on the part of the agricultural industry to chemically alter what Nature has provided. It would seem that Man knows more than Nature; even some scientists live with this illusion. The whole basis for the chemical manipulation of food is to make money. There is no regard for the animal or for the consumer. It's portrayed as being of benefit to you, the consumer, but nothing could be further from the truth. It's about dollars, euros and pounds.

As if enough damage hasn't already been done to the soil and to milk, cows need to be made more productive, so they have now become the next source of interference. The aim now is to hormonally interfere with the dairy herds so that they yield more milk so that the supermarkets and middlemen make more money. In the past 50 years, dairy farming has been changed from a very natural process into an industrial-scale operation. Cows are now producing double the volume of milk on average than they were 50 years ago. This is because of the use of hormones and artificial feed. A single cow has only a limited supply of minerals, vitamins, essential fats, etc. If the output of milk has doubled, then the nutrient level of the milk has halved. We are producing more milk than ever before, but of poor quality. The ultimate effect of this is to weaken the health of both animals and consumers. Again, there is no wisdom or respect in evidence. The free market is free to damage the entire ecosystem that we call Earth, or so it would appear. Leadership is sadly lacking. Money controls politicians and other leaders in the society. They have been rendered powerless to protect you and me. It's time to take back control ourselves.

You can't feed cows industrial grains and expect a good outcome. Cows need to be kept outside in the open air and feed on natural pastures containing a mixture of grasses, flowers and herbs. This is the most humane way to raise the animal; only then will you get good-quality milk. It's inhumane to keep cattle in sheds all year round and feed them unnatural foods such as genetically modified cereals and meat-and-bone meal. This has led to the development of mad cow disease and its human equivalent, Creutzfeldt-Jakob disease. In essence, you're supporting this type of farming and endorsing the inhumane treatment of animals when you purchase pasteurised milk from your supermarket. You're also getting a far inferior product compared to organic milk or raw milk direct from the farmer. If you would prefer not to use dairy milk at all, then use another, less commercial source of milk, such as goat or sheep milk.

Farming is now effectively controlled by chemical companies that are destroying the environment and producing not just poor-quality food, but toxic food. Food manufacturers are more interested in quantity than quality. They make such huge profits from the sale of processed foods that they can afford to bribe politicians, doctors and dieticians. Cows are now being farmed to produce more milk via the use of hormones such as growth hormone and through the use of genetically modified cereals such as soya. It is high time for people to rebel and for traditional farming methods to return.

Chapter 7
Breaking the Supermarket Habit

INTRODUCTION

The purpose of this chapter is to alert you to the toxins in food items you may consider harmless and thereby help to wean you off the dependence on the weekly shop in the supermarket. This is not to say you have to avoid the supermarket completely, but rather be more selective in what you buy there. It will also make you more political in nature and much less accepting of the status quo: more political in that you will be much more aware of the games being played by the food companies and of the link these companies have with advisory bodies and less accepting of the status quo in that you won't be as trusting of advisory bodies or of any authority figure or organisation in society, but more trusting of your own instincts. Let's first examine some of the most dangerous toxins in common food items.

TOXINS IN COMMON FOODS

Artificial sweeteners

What if I told you there was a substance in your diet and in your children's diet that has been shown to cause malignant brain tumours in experimental animals? What if I told you this same substance was rejected three times by the US Food and Drug Administration (FDA) between 1975 and 1980? What if I told you that the FDA accused the company that manufactures this substance of scientific fraud because important evidence about the experiments done on laboratory animals was withheld and data was deliberately manipulated, and as a consequence the case was referred to the Attorney General's office in Washington? What if I told you that when President Reagan came to power in 1980 he removed the commissioner of the FDA and replaced him with a new one, Dr Hayes, who approved the same substance, and that two years later Dr Hayes was forced to resign amid a corruption scandal? What if I told you that many scientists and doctors are calling for a reappraisal of this substance as the incidence of brain tumours in adults and children increases?

The substance I'm speaking about is aspartame (trade name NutraSweet or Equal). It's the most popular artificial sweetener and is used in a variety of food items and beverages as well as a number of tablets, including children's vitamin tablets. Chances are you have consumed this substance on a number of occasions. It's mainly found in diet drinks such as Diet Coke or Diet 7Up but has increasingly been used in children's medicines and in a lot of cold and flu remedies.

Aspartame was discovered by accident in a laboratory in Chicago in 1965. The chemist who discovered it was employed by G.D. Searle, a pharmaceutical company, to work on the development of a new anti-ulcer drug. He realised that the substance that he had made by combining two amino acids together was very, very sweet – in fact, 200 times sweeter than table sugar. The company decided to do research on it over the coming years and applied for approval from the FDA. Three applications were made between 1975 and 1980 and three times it was rejected.

The rejections were centred around the fact that aspartame was shown to have caused various tumours in laboratory animals (Stoddard, 1998). Aspartame was shown to have caused brain tumours, pancreatic tumours, breast tumours and uterine tumours. One of the by-products of aspartame metabolism is a chemical called diketopiperazine (DKP), which is known to be carcinogenic. This is the chemical that the FDA was most concerned about, and rightly so. But it is not just the production of this chemical that is of concern.

Aspartame is quite a simple substance, composed of two amino acids that form part of everyone's diet. These two amino acids are found in all meat that you eat, such as steak. So what's the problem with consuming them in high quantities in aspartame, you might ask? Lots of professional athletes use high-protein shakes and amino acid supplements for years with apparently no ill effects. Surely the fact that aspartame is approved in over 90 countries is sufficient evidence that it's safe for human consumption. After all, the experiments were done on rats, not humans, and it's hard to make definitive statements based on this evidence.

It's not the two amino acids in aspartame that are so toxic, it's the chemical that binds the two amino acids together. This chemical is converted in the body to methanol, which is poisonous to humans. Methanol has killed many alcoholics over the years. The reason why it's so poisonous is because it's converted to formaldehyde, which is used to preserve dead bodies, organs, etc. in laboratories. It has a very pungent odour and really stinks. I remember it well from anatomy dissection rooms; it used to make me feel nauseous every time we had to do dissections. Formaldehyde is toxic to the nervous system and creates a whole array of symptoms, as the following case history illustrates.

Mary was in her late twenties when she came to see me a few years ago complaining of severe early morning head-ache. She woke every day with a severe headache that eased during the day but never went away. The headache had been present for over two years and it was slowly wearing her down. She was becoming quite depressed as a consequence and her workmates found her more moody and irritable. She also found that her vision was being affected, as words on the page were becoming blurred. She had tried all kind of painkillers and other drugs and had experimented with all kinds of diets, but to no avail. She had been investigated by a neurologist and her brain scan and other tests were all normal. I sensed the cause of her headache was somewhat unusual, as all the tests that I did, including toxicity tests, were also normal.

It was only after the exclusion of individual chemicals in her diet that progress was made. It wasn't just aspartame that was causing her headache, but all the artificial sweet-eners, including saccharine and acesulfame K. When we excluded all these artificial sweeteners, her headache was 50 per cent better. What was causing the remainder? It turned out to be monosodium glutamate (MSG), which is used to enhance the flavour of a lot of foods – she loved Chinese food and flavoured crisps. When she excluded MSG as well, her headaches disappeared within a few days, as did all her other symptoms.

Headaches are the least of your worries where the consumption of aspartame is concerned. A study published in the *American Journal of Clinical Nutrition* in December 2012 showed a link between aspartame consumption and blood cancers such as lymphoma, multiple myeloma and leukaemia (Schernhammer et al., 2012). Other studies have also confirmed the cancer-forming ability of aspartame (Soffritti, 2007 et al.; Whetsell, 1996).

Unfortunately, such a message would embarrass the government, the FDA and bring many lawsuits against the major food companies in the US, so the message had to be altered to say that 'further research needs to be done'. This study was funded by the National Institutes of Health and the National Cancer Institute with public money. The study is the only one to date that has looked at long-term exposure to aspartame and at a large number of people. The study lasted 22 years and had 48,000 male and 77,000 female participants. Each participant drank more than one diet soda drink per day. The results showed a higher incidence of leukaemia than one would expect and a higher incidence of lymphoma and multiple myeloma (both blood cancers). The leukaemia occurred in both sexes, but the lymphoma and myeloma were found only in males. The authors could not explain this strange finding. The study was faultless and thus stands up to scientific and medical scrutiny. It's the most important study done to date on artificial sweeteners. It involved humans, not experimental animals, and so can be used to deliver a powerful message about the harm these chemicals are having on the health of people worldwide.

However, now that you know that the tail wags the dog in the us and that the food companies tell politicians, Harvard Medical School and many of the advisory bodies in the us as well as international bodies such as the World Health Organization what to say, you will never hear the truth. I predict that the food companies will now sponsor research to conflict with this study so as to create controversy. That has been their ploy for years and was the ploy of the tobacco industry a few decades ago.

We have known since the 1970s about the link between consumption of aspartame and brain tumours in laboratory rats. We did not know there was any link between consuming more than one can of diet soda per day and blood cancers. This is why studies like this, which are funded with public money, are so important. You can now see that just because something has been approved by the FDA in the us or the Food Safety Authority in Ireland and the Food Standards Agency in the UK and is in the food chain doesn't necessarily make it safe to use. I suggest you put pressure on your local politician to have aspartame removed from the shelves. But before you do that, it's important to read on, as there may be additional things you may want removed from the food chain. Here are some of the commonly used tablets that contain aspartame:

- Vitamin tablets, such as Bugs Bunny and Flintstones multivitamin tablets
- Laxatives and bulking agents such as Maalox, Metamucil and Fybogel

- Antibiotics such as Augmentin and Amoxil
- Gut medicines such as Zantac, Pepcid and Zoton
- Respiratory medicines such as Singular and Benadryl
- Others such as Calcichew and Lemsip and Calpol for kids.

Sucralose

Sucralose is another artificial sweetener. It's made by adding a chlorine atom to sugar, which renders the molecule more sweet. It's sold under the trade name Splenda and was approved in 1991 by the FDA. It's found in many processed foods.

Duke University in the US did an interesting study on sucralose and found that it has significant adverse effects on the gut in particular (Abou-Donia et al., 2008). They found that using sucralose can reduce the good bacteria in your gut by up to 50 per cent. So if you're helping your body by taking a probiotic supplement or taking live yoghurt every day, this sweetener will undo a lot of your good work. The single most important protective effect against developing colon cancer is the bacterial flora of the gut.

This sweetener also disturbs the gut's pH balance. It makes the stomach less acidic, thus impairing the digestion of protein, and it makes the small intestine less alkaline, thus impairing the digestion of all other foods. This is very significant, as anything that interferes with digestion means the nutrients are less available for absorption, so you don't gain the benefit of what you're eating.

A study reported in the *Canadian Journal of Gastroenterology* suggested that sucralose in particular may be the reason why colitis and Crohn's disease (inflammatory bowel disease, IBD) have become more common of late in Canada (Qin et al., 2011).

Early studies done on IBD showed that the disease was more prevalent in the UK, Scandinavia and the US (Qin et al., 2011). These countries always topped the list. Yet a more recent study has shown Canada as top of the list (Qin et al., 2011). Doctors in Canada were at a loss to explain this and began to examine food additives that had adverse effects on the gut. They found that the incidence of IBD in Alberta province in 1981 was 44 per 100,000 of the population. By the year 2000, this had risen to 283 per 100,000 of the population. The incidence of IBD was over six times higher in the space of 20 years. The doctors knew it had to be something in the food chain causing this. They looked at all the possible additives that could cause this and isolated sucralose as the most likely culprit.

This study is corroborated by another study recently published in the *World Journal of Gastroenterology*. In this study, carried out by Dr Qin of New Jersey Medical School in the US, there is clear evidence of a link between the introduction of sucralose and a rise in the incidence of IBD (Qin et al., 2012). He suggests that IBD is caused by saccharin and sucralose. When the use of saccharin declined in the late 1970s because of cancer scares, the rate of IBD also declined. In countries where sucralose (Splenda) was approved, the incidence of IBD increased, as was the case in Canada. Dr Qin suggests that both artificial sweeteners damage the gut flora and in so doing damage gut function. After 12 weeks of taking Splenda, the levels of *bifidobacterium* and *lactobacilli* are significantly reduced. These two species of bacteria are the very ones doctors use to treat IBD.

Sucralose, or Splenda, is found in a whole host of foods: breakfast cereals, drinks, desserts, toppings, fillings, chewing gum, jams, salad creams, biscuits and cakes. It has been approved by the FSA and the FDA. Because of the increased risk of developing IBD and therefore an increased risk of developing colon cancer (people with IBD have a higher risk of developing cancer), it's best to avoid not just sucralose and saccharin, but all artificial sweeteners.

The common reactions from taking it include abdominal symptoms such as bloating, wind, cramps and diarrhoea, sometimes with blood in it. Other symptoms include skin reactions such as peeling, blisters, crusting, itchiness and hives and central nervous system symptoms such as headache, migraine, impaired concentration, depression and anxiety. In the lungs it can cause shortness of breath, wheezing and cough. If you have any of these symptoms, avoid artificial sweeteners. Often artificial sweeteners are combined to produce the desired level of sweetness. All of these sweeteners have been associated with various cancers in experimental animals or in humans.

Another sweetener, acesulfame K, is commonly added to soft drinks and foodstuffs, yet it contains methylene chloride, a known carcinogen. Experimental studies done on laboratory animals have shown that it can cause multiple tumours, e.g. breast tumours, thyroid tumours and blood tumours (Jacobsen, Lefferts and Garland, 1993). The question one must ask is why are such seriously dangerous chemicals in our food? And who allowed this to happen?

The argument for including them is that no long-term studies have been done to establish their safety, with the exception of the study carried out by Brigham and Women's Hospital mentioned above (Schernhammer et al., 2012).

Most of the studies submitted to the FDA and FSA are short-term studies done over weeks, not years. Also, it's difficult to extrapolate information gained from experimental studies done on animals to the human population. The argument against including them is pretty obvious: if there is the slightest risk of doing harm to people, they must be banned until long-term studies have proven they are safe.

You're now beginning to learn where the huge increase in the incidence of various cancers in Western society is coming from. The WHO has admitted publicly that most cancers are dietary related. Why, then, don't we hear public bodies advising people to avoid processed food? Food companies are putting carcinogens into your food and getting away with it.

Butylated hydroxyanisole (BHA)

BHA is a chemical added to various foods to prevent the fat or oil in the food from going rancid. In other words, it delays the oxidation of fats, giving the food a longer shelf life. It's added in small quantities and was thought to be quite safe; it's added in bigger quantities to a number of medicines, some of which you may know as statins, which lower cholesterol.

There appears to be a lot of controversy surrounding the use of BHA. Some authorities say it's safe, while others are suggesting it's a potential carcinogen. (Here we go again, I hear you say.) The FDA in America says it has GRAS status, which means it is 'generally regarded as safe'. However, the National Institutes of Health (NIH) says it's 'reasonably anticipated to be a carcinogen'. The reason why the NIH says this is because in high doses it has been shown to cause cancer in rats, mice and hamsters, albeit in the fore stomach, which humans don't have. The International Agency for Research on Cancer labels it as a possible human carcinogen. Canada has flagged BHA as a 'high human health priority' and will review all the evidence regarding it more closely.

If you were a member of the FSA or FDA, would you approve the use of such a substance? For years, bodies such as the FSA and FDA have argued that just because a food chemical is carcinogenic in animals doesn't mean it's carcinogenic in humans. This is the argument that has been presented to endorse the use of aspartame, which in the recent Brigham and Women's Hospital study has been shown to cause leukaemia in humans.

Which foods do you find BHA in? In potato crisps (called 'potato chips' in some countries), butter, cereal, instant mashed potato, processed meats, beer, baked goods, dessert mixes, chewing gum, pastries and some sauces, to name a few. Read the label of any processed food. BHA is also found in a number of cosmetics, such as lipsticks and moisturisers. It has the potential to cause severe allergic skin reactions and has been banned by the European Union for use in cosmetics.

Its cousin, butylated hydroxytoluene (BHT), which is also used to preserve fats and can be found in the same foods, medicines and cosmetics mentioned above, has also been flagged as a risk by many authorities, as it has been shown to cause liver, thyroid and kidney problems as well as disrupting hormones in the body. Canada has also flagged it, but as a 'moderate human health priority'.

Because this is already on many people's list as a potential carcinogen and because it can cause damage to a number of organs, you should avoid BHT. It should be banned in any product for human use. Then, and only then, it should be thoroughly investigated.

I have listed only a small number of chemicals that are of concern in the foods that you eat – aspartame, sucralose, acesulfame K and the fat preservatives BHA and BHT – to warn you to consider what you're buying very seriously. I have also tried to help you see how unprotected you are by the protection agencies such as the FSA and the FDA. I'm also arguing that the increasing incidence of many cancers in the Western world has everything to do with what you're putting into your body, especially foodstuffs and beverages.

A lot of cancer research has to do with finding new modes of treatment, mainly drug treatments, and very little to do with diet. There is no money for doctors or the drug companies in telling you to avoid certain foods; there is a lot of money, however, in cancer treatment. Preventative medicine is the key but gets little mention in medical education or in universities. I foresee that as the drug companies decline, nutritional medicine will come to the fore as the main form of treatment not only for cancer, but for a whole host of medical complaints. Nutritional medicine is the future.

BREAKING THE HABIT

You, the consumer, are misinformed and often very confused because of conflicting advice. The farmer has been hijacked by the chemical companies, while the food companies make millions from feeding you toxic foods.

Supermarkets control approximately 80 per cent of the grocery trade in the British Isles, so in essence they control to a great extent what we eat and thus control our level of health.

Start looking at the supermarket as a health (or nutritional) clinic that sells you medicine to make your body healthy. If you have a cold or flu, they will sell you fresh lemons and oranges. If you have arthritis, they will encourage you to buy brightly coloured vegetables, and so on. Then, when you see foods that will make you sick, such as processed foods, you will be scared to eat them in the same way that you would be scared to take medicine that wasn't prescribed for you. They will provide the medicine you require, so ask for organic meat that is produced locally, ask for organically grown vegetables and fruits produced locally, ask for lots of fresh, wild seafood and ask for cereals that have not been sprayed with chemicals and are not genetically modified. The use of local produce helps everyone in that it's more likely to be fresh and transport costs are reduced. Supermarkets need you to take control and make demands either individually or as a group. Supermarkets are sensitive to consumer demands.

The truth about supermarkets is that at present, they provide foods that suit them first and foremost. They like foods that have a long shelf life and can be transported with minimal spoilage. They also prefer large-scale production to ensure regular supplies and maximum profit. You have the power to change all that. When you do your weekly shopping, you're involved in the single most important act regarding the health not just of your family, but of the whole nation. By supporting good eating habits such as buying only organic produce and by refusing processed foods, you are changing the face of Western civilisation.

The manufacturers of processed foods, such as Coca-Cola, PepsiCo, Kellogg's, Danone, Mars, Nestlé, etc., will go into decline and eventually go out of business. The demand for real farm produce, organically produced, will reduce the power of the chemical companies and eventually they will disappear as well and farmers will be able to grow food the old-fashioned way. That way, you can be sure the soil is no longer being destroyed and will regenerate. By refusing to support the manufacturers of processed food, you are also diminishing their power over the medical profession, over politicians, over advisory bodies such as the FSA and FDA and over world bodies such as the WHO.

You can see that your simple act of grocery shopping has enormous consequences for your whole society. So how do you break the supermarket habit? It's simply about changing your mindset before you enter the shop.

Think health, not food; think building blocks for the body, not satisfying your cravings; think boundless energy, not tiredness and lethargy. When making your shopping list, include the following:

- Safe water
- Good bacteria
- Fats and oils
- Protein
- Minerals
- Vitamins
- Starch
- A few treats.

Under safe water, try to buy your water in a glass bottle, such as San Pellegrino, or if you can't find that, then buy Spa, Volvic or Isklar water. If you have a filter at home such as a reverse osmosis filter, then you don't need to buy bottled water. Also, buy yourself a present of a total dissolved solids (TDS) meter, which will tell you how pure your water is. You can purchase one online (such as www.tdsmeter.com) or you can get it from companies that supply instruments for science laboratories in schools and universities.

To get good bacteria, the best option is to make your own yoghurt at home. Yoghurt makers are available on the internet (such as www.lakeland.co.uk) or any shop that sells kitchenware. If you don't have the time to make your own or don't want to, then buy a plain natural yoghurt with no added sugar and also buy a probiotic supplement in the health shop. Open the capsule and add a little of the contents to the yoghurt and leave it at room temperature overnight. Take the yoghurt on an empty stomach and wait before putting hot liquids such as tea into your stomach. Give the bacteria time to multiply and pass through the gut before eating breakfast. There are good live yoghurts available in supermarkets, but they are best bought in health shops, farm shops or farmers' markets where you can be sure you're getting the real deal.

Fats and oils would include some of the following: fat for frying food, fat for baking, oil for cooking and foods containing healthy fats. When frying meats, for example, always use butter or lard (pork fat), as they are more stable at high temperatures. The best fat for baking is unquestionably lard, which most good chefs are now reverting back to. Use extra virgin olive oil if cooking on low to medium heat. Avoid all other commercial oils, such as sunflower, sesame, corn or rapeseed oils. Buy foods that are rich in essential fats and in cholesterol. Buy lots of free-range hen and duck eggs, organic bacon, organic beef with the fat attached, etc. Animal fat is essential for energy and for the cell membranes. Because a lot of people are deficient in omega 3 oils, buy fish oil or flaxseed oil or ground-up flaxseeds, such as Virginia Harvest brand, instead.

The best protein is animal protein, as it has all 22 amino acids. Eat lots of lambs liver when available and other organ meats such as kidney and heart. Also eat free-range chicken and organic beef and pork. If you don't like animal produce, then eat lots of vegetable protein but combine the proteins so that you have the full complement of amino acids. The best protein and the most easily digested one is fish, but it should be fresh and caught out at sea, not farmed.

Minerals come from the soil. If the soil isn't deficient, you should be able to get a good supply of minerals from animals that feed on natural pastures. For example, dairy is important, but try to get raw milk; if you can't, try to buy organic. Try to trace the local producer of the organic milk and see if the farmer will supply you with raw milk. Supermarkets these days will bamboozle you with the many types of milk available, such as whole milk, low-fat milk, semi-skimmed milk, skimmed milk, etc., so you have to be prepared before you enter and focus only on what you want. Avoid all processed cheese because of the possible cancer risk mentioned above and only buy unprocessed cheese from a farm shop or farmers' market.

Buy lots of fresh, organic vegetables and lots of organic fruits. Make juices at home and only cook vegetables lightly. Buy lots of ingredients to make simple salads. Use olive oil and lemon juice as a dressing. Buy lemons and add them to tea and to carbonated water. Take a glass of lukewarm water with the juice of one lemon each morning before breakfast. It's best to eat fruits and vegetables in season.

Cereals such as wheat, rye, oats, barley, maize, millet, etc. are generally a problem for a variety of reasons. Suffice it to say that if you want to use them, try to use organically grown cereals and pre-digest them, such as soaking them overnight, as I have mentioned earlier in this book. If you're Celtic in origin and have digestive problems, it's best to avoid all cereals or use them infrequently.

The best source of B vitamins is yeast, so use foods that contain yeast, such as wine or beer. Your supply of other vitamins will come from the fats you eat and the fruit and vegetables. Because vitamin C is not stored in the body, top up your supply in the winter months, as fruits rich in vitamin C are scarce at this time of year and so you have a greater risk of viral infections such as colds and flu.

There's no harm in an occasional treat. I have a weakness for apple pie and feel the need to treat myself every so often. It's not what you're doing infrequently that matters, but rather what you're eating daily. Obviously if you have an addiction to a particular food you'll have to avoid it completely; otherwise, enjoy the odd treat, whatever that means to you.

GOLDEN RULES FOR GROCERY SHOPPING

1. **No children:** When doing your weekly shopping, the first golden rule is to leave the kids at home, with a relative or in a crèche in the shopping centre – do not bring them with you. A lot of adverts for new breakfast cereals, cereal bars and soft drinks are directed at young children who put their

parents under pressure to buy these products. When you do the shopping there's no harm in a few treats for you and your family. Just be selective in what you are calling a treat.

2. **Use a basket or small trolley:** The second golden rule is to use a small trolley or a basket to limit what you buy. Alternatively, shop online – that way, you don't have to load and unload items a few times and you don't have to drop off and collect children.

3. **Be very focused:** Don't get distracted by special offers, good deals and other marketing ploys. Know what you want before you enter and wear blinkers until you find what you're looking for.

4. **Ask a lot of questions:** For example, ask how fresh the vegetables and fruits are, ask where the bacon or meat or fish or chicken has come from and take the name and contact details of the farmers, etc. It's best to ask for the manager and make a list of questions for him or her.

FARMERS' MARKETS, FARM SHOPS AND BOX SCHEMES

There is a gradually expanding interest in farmers' markets in Ireland and the UK. Almost one-third of the population prefers to buy produce directly from the farmer because of the lack of middlemen and because they can ask questions and get straight answers (Harvey, 2008). The human interaction in the process of buying what are critically important items for your well-being is very important; you are much more likely to buy from someone with whom you have had a positive interaction and whom you believe to be honest and trustworthy. People are fed up with being conned by adverts, posters, sponsorship of events, etc. They can get a feel for the person selling the produce, ask as many questions as they wish and then test the goods at home. A farmer who sells directly to neighbours, friends and the local community is much more likely to take greater care over the production of their food than a farmer who sells produce to a food manufacturer or to a meat factory. The farmer's reputation is at stake, so you're more likely to get a better deal.

The nice thing about farmers' markets is that there are two simple rules governing them. Firstly, the food has to be produced locally, normally within a certain radius of the market. Secondly, the seller must be familiar with the production process so that they are able to field all manner of questions. Some people find these markets a bit more expensive than the local supermarket, which is true, but it's about the quality of the produce, which is well worth the extra cost, and it's about avoiding illness, which can be very costly.

The number of farmers' markets in both the UK and Ireland is growing rapidly. The first one in the UK opened in 1997 in the West Country; today, there are approximately 500. In Ireland the first one began in Dublin; today, there are almost 10 operating in and around Dublin. In addition, many towns have a local market once a week. By supporting these farmers' markets, you're supporting a revolution in the way food is produced and sold. You're supporting good farming practices and traditional methods of farming and reconnecting people with the farmers. This interface between eater and producer is of profound importance, not only because you get better and safer produce, but because the surface of our planet doesn't get damaged any further by industrial farming methods.

Farm shops are an even better idea, as you're more likely to see the animals face to face, so to speak, and can inspect the fields on which produce is grown. It's important to see the animals on a farm because one can tell a lot about what happens on the farm by inspecting the livestock. For example, are the hens or ducks allowed to wander freely around the fields and are the cattle alert, but quiet? Also, are there flowers and herbs growing in the fields, as natural pastures will have different types of grasses, herbs and flowers in the same field? You can tell much by merely visiting a farm shop.

The farmer in this instance is hardly likely to attract customers if his or her farm is run badly, so the presence of a farm shop is automatically a good sign. If someone in the shop is willing to show you around the farm, then or at some future point in time, this is also a very good sign. However, not all the produce in a farm shop may come from the one farm. Neighbouring farmers may sell their produce through this one outlet. But since it's a neighbour, it's relatively easy to cast an eye over their farm as well. Life-long relationships are made by visiting farms, because if you're happy with the produce, you won't want to buy from anywhere else. You will be able to revert back in time and be able to eat wholesome, natural foods, as I was lucky enough to do when I was a child.

Box schemes are yet another way of getting good produce if you don't wish to visit a local farmers' market or farm shop. Where I live there is a local producer of organically grown vegetables who supplies a range of vegetables delivered in a box to my home. This is an excellent way of getting deliveries of fruits and vegetables.

The other main way of accessing good produce is to use the internet. Search for 'organic produce' or 'organic farmers' and you will find a host of useful information. Useful websites are as follows:

- www.irishfarmersmarkets.ie
- www.iofga.org
- www.living-organically.com
- www.alotoforganics.co.uk

The Irish Organic Farmers and Growers Association (IOFGA) has a directory of members and can put you in touch with a farmer or grower close to where you live. Log on to their website (www.iofga.org) for contact details.

FINAL NOTE

Hopefully you now have some basic information to start feeding yourself and your family well. If you give yourself time, you'll be able to wean yourself away from the supermarket. It's a matter of taking time to source alternative suppliers of basic food items, making sure the produce from these outlets is of good quality and making sure that the price is right for you. It's good to shop in the same place to give time for people to get to know you and what your tastes are. All prices are negotiable, but wait for the people in the shop to realise that you're a regular customer and then they'll be more flexible on price. As time progresses, spend less in the supermarket and more on **good food**.

Chapter 8
What Is Good Food?

INTRODUCTION

What is good food? It's a simple and important question to ask, but the answer is somewhat complicated. When I began to write this book it was my intention to deal with simple concepts like listing the key foods, including water, and then discussing each of these in turn and comparing older methods of cooking with modern methods. But the more I thought about it, the broader the topic became. I quickly realised that I had to write about much more than processed foods compared to natural foods. I was also acutely aware that I had to keep things simple and easy to read, which is sometimes quite hard to do.

I realised that good food comes from healthy plants and animals, which in turn come from a healthy soil, which in turn is highly dependent on farming methods. Although I grew up in the countryside in Northern Ireland and lived amongst the farming community, I knew little about farming. In researching farming methods, I essentially had to rewrite this book to include a very important story not just about modern farming methods, but about the increasing political control of food production since the 1940s.

That research led me back to what makes a soil healthy, which in turn led me back to the creation of the planet and the creation of all the essential elements (carbon, hydrogen, oxygen, nitrogen, calcium, magnesium, etc.) that create life. It led me back to the creation of the universe and how dependent we are not just on the planet we live on, but on the whole universe. We are not only linked to other living creatures, but we are also totally dependent on rocks being eroded to release minerals to feed the soil. These rocks (and thus you too) ultimately come from outer space. All the chemical elements in the periodic table that you may have learned about in science class at school are manufactured deep in space in dying stars. For example, carbon, which forms the basis of all organic foodstuffs, is made far beyond this planet. Iron, which carries oxygen around your body, is an element formed in deep space. All life as we know it began in the furnace of dying stars. Dying stars form the whole chemistry set of life.

The topic of good food spreads its tentacles far beyond cooking methods, food processing, farming methods and soil analysis into the murky world of politics, corruption and the genetic modification of seeds. In truth, the topic of good food is so broad that it requires a number of books. What I have decided to do in this book is to give you an overview but also to inform and alert you to some important issues.

ORGANIC FARMING

I begin this chapter with a positive story. In 1996 Jody Scheckter, former winner of the Formula One World Drivers' Championship, bought a farm in Hampshire, about 40 miles from London. Growing up in East London, South Africa, and being a professional race car driver taught Jody the importance of good food to keep his body in peak condition. Being married with young children, his aim was to set up a farm that could produce the best food possible for him and his family. His aim was simply to learn how to produce healthy food. He was aware that nutrition was going to become the most important issue in the years ahead.

He bought 2,500 acres of land near Basingstoke and proceeded to learn everything possible about farming. He soon realised that his farm had to be organic, free from all chemical fertilisers and pesticides, and that traditional methods would have to be used to improve the quality of the food. Quoting from his website (www.laverstokepark.co.uk), he said, 'Ninety per cent of farming is soil.' To guarantee a good-quality soil he set up his own soil analysis laboratory with the ultimate in high-tech equipment. A lot of time, energy and money have gone into improving both the mineral content of the soil and its microbial content. Microbes such as bacteria and fungi convert inorganic minerals into organic minerals that plants can absorb and use.

He is also adamant that a large number of grasses, seeds, herbs and clover are used at planting time. The more varied the species of plants growing on these natural pastures, the richer the quality of produce. He endorses the principle of biodiversity, saying that it produces high-quality pastures for his livestock to feed on. The milk from his cattle and buffalo has higher levels of fat-soluble vitamins (A, D, E and K) and conjugated linoleic acid (CLA), which is a proven anti-cancer substance. What Jody says is indeed borne out by scientific research. Modern research has shown that foods from livestock fed on natural pastures have high levels of omega 3 oils and high levels of fat-soluble vitamins (Daley, 2010).

He is passionate about his farm and insists on slow-growing

pastures and slow-growing livestock. Hence, he prefers Jersey dairy cows over the high-yielding Holsteins that are commonly used on other dairy farms in the British Isles. He also produces buffalo milk, which is much creamier than cow milk and suitable for making ice cream.

What's interesting is that he prefers to sell directly to the consumer. However, since he has a massive volume of produce he also sells to supermarkets such as Waitrose. He produces milk, cheese, yoghurt, ice cream and butter as well as beef, buffalo meat, lamb, chicken, turkey, pork and free-range eggs. Add to that some of the best-tasting fruits and vegetables and you'll be left in no doubt as to just how good food can actually be. What I like about what he has done is that he has set up a powerful example of how successful natural methods of farming can be. His produce is out of this world and is in great demand by top chefs in the UK. He does indeed produce good food for his family and for the wider community. He has set an example for other farmers and for all of us who are passionate about good nutrition.

In Ireland there is another good example of organic farming set in the hills of west Wicklow close to the town of Ballymore Eustace. It's called Ballymore Farm and produces a range of organic dairy produce, including raw milk, buttermilk, butter, cream and yoghurt. Like Jody Scheckter, Aidan Harney and his partner, Mary, prefer Jersey and Ayrshire cows and natural pastures with many species of grass, herbs, flowers and clover. They have 70 cows in all and supply a range of outlets in Dublin, Wicklow and Kildare as well as selling fresh produce in farmers' markets and also directly to the consumer via a shop on their farm.

However, good food isn't defined by Jody Scheckter or Aidan Harney; it's defined by Nature. Good food doesn't only come from organic or biodynamic farms. It can come from the simplest of places, such as an allotment close to your town or city or even your own back garden. How, then, can you distinguish between something rich in nutrients and something that is not? With regard to fruit and vegetables, there are ways to tell.

Firstly, there's the taste test. Buy a range of fruit or vegetables from a number of shops and supermarkets. Rank them on a scale of zero to 10, where zero represents no taste and 10 represents produce that's sweet and juicy. You will be amazed by the range of scores. Choose one fruit to begin with, e.g. apples, and get the whole family involved. Then compare your scores.

Secondly, buy or borrow an instrument called a Brix refractometer. This simple-to-use and inexpensive device will tell you if the fruit is ripe. It has helped wine growers around the world to decide the correct time to harvest their grapes. It can now be used to measure the ripeness of all fruits and vegetables. Just extract a drop or two of the juice, place it on a slide and insert it into the device. A fruit or vegetable grown on poor soil will give a low reading, whereas one grown on good soil will have a much higher reading. The device measures the solid content of the juice; in other words, it measures the sugar, vitamin and mineral content of the juice. A high sugar level indicates ripeness and a high vitamin and mineral content indicates a rich soil, so the higher the reading, the better.

Armed with a Brix refractometer, go round shops and farm shops, farmers' markets and supermarkets and test the nutritional value of what's on offer. It's a powerful way to get children interested in nutrition and would make a great teaching tool for schools. Buy a basic one for about €50, as the more sophisticated ones are for industry and research and big businesses such as wine growing.

What you may discover from this simple experiment will likely alarm you. The majority of the fresh produce sold in cities and towns is of poor quality. Experiments performed across the world with this device show two patterns (Harrill, 1994). Firstly, most fruit and vegetables are grown on poor soils – over 70 per cent in developed countries such as the UK, US and Canada. Secondly, there's a wide variety in the quality, such that one box of apples may have a mixture of good-quality, medium-quality and poor-quality fruit. The fruit and vegetables that show a high reading on the refractometer will invariably deliver high-quality nutrients and will taste good too.

It's also interesting to compare organically grown produce with non-organic produce. One would suspect that the former would be superior in quality, and generally this is the case. However, it depends on the soil in which the fruit is grown. If the quality of the soil is poor, then the quality of the produce will be poor irrespective of the method of farming. Thus, organically grown produce is not necessarily of superior quality, but in many cases it is. Quality is ultimately dependent on the mineral and microbial content of the soil. As Jody Scheckter says, 'farming is 90 per cent soil'. That's why he has a laboratory to analyse the minerals in soil and a separate laboratory to measure the microbial content of the soil.

But just because a soil is in its natural state and hasn't been exposed to artificial fertilisers and chemical sprays doesn't mean the soil will produce good crops – far from it, in fact. The soil may be deficient in earthworms or essential bacteria or minerals. Sandy soils may be deficient in copper, while chalk or limestone soils can be deficient in manganese. It's necessary to test the soil regularly. If the soil is deficient in certain minerals, it's important to dress the soil with minerals. The best source of minerals comes from ground-up rocks, also called rock dust.

Traditionally, farmers used plant and animal waste as a source of minerals and as a source of organic waste for the microbial content of the soil to feed on. Where I grew up in Northern Ireland, farmers used animal dung as a natural fertiliser. It enriched the soil but did little to uplift the community. These farmers also used chalk or limestone dressings, as these are rich in calcium. In the early 1900s farmers across Europe used basic slag, which is a by-product of steel making, as it was rich in minerals such as iron, zinc, copper and manganese. However, the onset of the Second World War and the introduction of artificial fertilisers changed farming completely (see Chapter 6 for more on this).

The mineralisation of soil has to do with the erosion of rocks. Minerals such as iron are made deep in outer space. These minerals are then blown across the universe as a star dies and explodes. These remnants of the dying star form a dust and eventually clump together to form rocks as the temperature drops. These rocks coalesce to form bigger rocks and ultimately asteroids and planets. The planet we live on is really a huge rock laden with minerals. When rock is ground down by erosion to form a powder or dust, the minerals are released. Microbes can then convert these minerals into a form that plants can use. For example, adding calcium to a soil allows bacteria in the soil to convert this inorganic mineral to calcium phosphate, which is an organic molecule that is accessible to the plant. Minerals can only be absorbed and utilised by the plant in their organic form. Now you can see why microbes are so important: they help plants to grow by converting all minerals to a user-friendly form. If you want to grow fantastic crops, fruits and vegetables, the magic lies in the microbes and a supply of minerals.

There is a magical place in the hills of southern Scotland called the Sustainable Ecological Earth Regeneration Centre (SEER Centre). It's a centre dedicated to the remineralisation of soil damaged by years of artificial fertilisers and chemical sprays. The centre produces rock dust and sells it across the UK to help farmers and gardeners regenerate their soil. The centre is run by Cameron and Moira Thomson, who have done experiments with the rock dust in their own garden. They ploughed up their quarter-acre garden and added lots of rock dust as well as organic waste. The result was amazingly big vegetables with an amazingly great taste. They then realised that this was possible on a much bigger scale and so set up the SEER Centre to teach people about the benefits of rock dust. Based on experiments they have carried out, they claim that using rock dust on a depleted soil not only improves the mineral content of the soil, but also improves soil structure and so increases its moisture-holding capacity. The plants get more water and air to the roots, allowing the plants to thrive.

The most important constituent of rock dust is silicon. Silicon strengthens the cell walls of the plant, which gives it the necessary strength to grow. Sandy soil has little available silicon and so is a poor soil on which to grow vegetables, but when rock dust is added it becomes much more fertile. Rock dust contains a range of minerals: calcium, magnesium, iron, sulphur, phosphorus, cobalt, copper, manganese, zinc and silicon. It can be spread on the soil by hand or with a spreader. It can then be mixed with the soil by hand or washed in with water. The amount to add to a soil depends on the quality of the soil to begin with. Poor soils may need as much as 10 to 20 tons per hectare. If you wish to learn more, look at the SEER website (www.seercentre.org.uk).

There's another benefit to using rock dust. The remineral-isation of soil not only produces healthier trees, plants, vegetables and fruits, but it also reduces the amount of carbon dioxide in the atmosphere. Growing plants need carbon dioxide and water to make food in a magical process called photosynthesis. Reducing atmospheric carbon dioxide levels will reduce global warming. Not only do you get great food, but you help the environment at the same time.

ENERGY LEVEL OF FOOD

Good food is much more than minerals and microbes, water and air, and a healthy soil; it is more than simply eating natural foods over processed foods; it is more than the pure physical value of food. Good food has emotional and spiritual energy as well. Eating food affects one's emotions, especially if the food has been prepared by a loved one such as a spouse, partner or parent. Sharing food strengthens the emotional bonds between people, which is why we invite friends to our home for a meal. Food connects people at a deeper level.

To explain the spiritual energy of food requires a visit to the cosmos again. The iron in your red blood cells that was formed far beyond this planet is really just an atom. Atoms, as you may already know, are composed mostly of energy and a small amount of matter in the nucleus. Even when the nucleus is split, it's found to be mostly energy as well. All the atoms making up your body are largely pure energy, which is collectively called your energy field. This energy field can be altered by the energy field of another human being, but it can also be altered by food. Food has the ability to affect your mood and your spirit in much the same way that anyone or anything else in your environment can.

At an individual level, food can affect your mood positively or negatively. In addition, the mood you're in has a direct relation to your choice of food. People who are emotionally upset or under a lot of stress tend to eat a lot of comfort foods such as sweet things, chocolate and starch in an attempt to quell the underlying emotion. What is perhaps not so well known is the effect that food can have on our emotions. I personally have experienced this when I was younger. When I ate sugary foods I used to wake up the next day feeling irritable and depressed. It took a few hours for this negative effect to lift. Sugary foods had a real and adverse effect on my emotional state of health. In some cases, this can set up a vicious cycle in that the worse you feel, the more you consume the wrong foods. The worse the level of stress or emotional upset, the worse your diet becomes. The energy of the food you're consuming reflects the emotions you're experiencing.

The opposite is also true. The more spiritual or aware you become, the less food you tend to eat and the more natural your diet becomes. Religion teaches us that we are a physical body with a soul. I prefer to see myself as a soul occupying a physical body for a short time. The essence or energy of your soul is reflected in your physical body. To allow this physical body to take you through life in a healthy state, start to regard it as sacred and the way in which you nourish it as sacred as well. The food you eat not only reflects your emotional state, but also where you're at in your relationship with your environment and with the planet. It reflects your spiritual awareness.

MINDFULNESS, GRATITUDE AND LOVE

When we're at peace with ourselves, we can devote our full attention to what we're doing. When we're in a relaxed state, we can focus on the food we most need to nourish ourselves and we can detect the effect that this food is having on us at all levels. To do this, we have to be fully present and aware of our intuition or gut feeling; we have to be in tune with our bodies. It's impossible to be in tune with your body when you're distracted with work, television, etc.

When eating in some countries in South America and Africa, one is taught to give thanks by offering a little food back to the earth. In the modern home, gratitude is often neglected. All food contains life and gives life to other creatures. To acknowledge this fact, it's important to say a prayer of gratitude, as it connects you to the rest of creation. Be grateful to have the chance to nourish your body and to have the energy to enjoy life. Plants and animals have been sacrificed to allow your life to continue.

Food is much more than purely satisfying a physical need. Food is 99 per cent energy and 1 per cent physical matter.

Focusing on the 1 per cent misses the whole purpose of food and of life. Rather, see everyone and everything as an energy field with which you will interact positively or negatively. Some foods will uplift you and make you feel good; others will pull you down and make you feel bad. Exactly the same can be said of people you meet. Looking at things from an energetic view-point will alter your awareness and you'll begin to see things in a very different way. You'll begin to see a whole new world.

The core of a child is love and the core of an adult is love. It's an energy that you feel but can't see or prove its existence. Love is the energy of the soul, and this is what connects people in very tight bonds. Out of love for his or her family, a parent will prepare food for everyone and look after all the physical needs of the family. It's often in the preparation and cooking of food that we see evidence of this love between family members. This is why it's important to involve children in the kitchen from an early age and why it's important for the whole family to sit and eat together.

LIVING FOOD VS. DEAD FOOD

Food connected to nature and not processed or altered chemically or physically should have all the substances needed to keep you alive and well. Most importantly, the energy of the food should be high enough to transmit that energy to you so that you can live life to the full and enjoy it thoroughly. Plants use light energy in a magical process called photosynthesis and pass on this energy either directly when you eat the plant or indirectly via grazing animals. This is another way in which we are connected to the universe. All life depends on the sun's energy via the process of photosynthesis. If plants stopped photosynthesizing, the rest of the living world would die. This daily need for energy connects us to the plants, which in turn are connected to the planet and to the sun. You are a link in an energy chain, so the food you eat should be viewed in this light.

Processing food alters the energy of the food. Exposing food to high temperatures and pressure (as in pasteurisation), squeezing it through machines (as in the extrusion of breakfast cereals), mixing it with dangerous chemicals (such as food additives) and exposing it to radiation (as with fruit, vegetables and spices) not only alters the energy field of the food, but can render it toxic to humans. These industrial processes can result in dead food that contains zero natural energy. In other words, the transfer of energy from the sun via plants and animals to us has been damaged; the energy chain is broken. Many processed foods that we consume, such as those found in tins, bottles, jars and packets, have such a low energy level that they have little value to the human body. Some of them are so altered that they can safely be defined as poisonous, such as those laden with sugar.

Many processed foods are stored in containers that can sufficiently lower the energy field of the food to render it unsafe. For example, when canned foods were first introduced, the cans were made of lead. The lead routinely leaked into the food and rendered it unsafe to eat. An example from today would be bottled water stored in plastic bottles. It's known that the chemicals in the plastic can leach into the water and render it toxic.

Good food is much more than its mere nutritional value, which everyone seems to focus on. Food is best viewed at an energy level. It's also important to recognise the emotional and spiritual value of food. By acknowledging the earth and giving thanks, you're acknowledging the work of the spiritual world to feed us and provide us with everything we need to stay healthy. Acknowledging that certain foods make you feel good connects you to yourself and to your emotions, which drive you.

Good food covers many areas of knowledge and expertise, from farming to healing. Good food connects you to me and to everyone else on the planet. It is the ultimate link in the chain of creation.

LESS IS MORE

The digestion, absorption and metabolism of food puts great demands on your body. It requires a lot of energy to break food down to its components and then for your liver to convert these components into energy. Even if the food is rich in nutrients and enzymes, it's still quite a process to metabolise the food; if the food is of poor quality or contains toxins such as food additives, the pressure on the liver is even greater. The secret of keeping your body healthy is to eat less.

The BBC programme *Horizon* investigated the diet of the inhabitants of the islands of Okinawa just south of Japan in an attempt to understand why they live so long and maintain such a high level of health. The average life expectancy is approximately 81 years, but many live well beyond that.

They analysed their diet and eating habits and discovered that they mostly ate fish and vegetables and restricted carbohydrates to a minimum. They also ate only when they were really hungry and ate only small meals. They never ate to the point of feeling a sense of fullness.

The idea of restricting carbohydrates to increase longevity isn't a new one. Experiments carried out in the 1930s in Cornell University in the US looked at the effects of calorie restriction on laboratory rats (Cousens, 2005). Their life expectancy doubled when their dietary calories were halved. Moreover, their level of health was much higher than the control rats on a normal diet. Since then, this experiment has been repeated a number of times by other researchers and confirmed.

Experiments done in the 1970s showed that even if you began a restricted calorie diet later in life, it had the desired effect of increasing longevity and improving the animals' level of health (Cousens, 2005). This has also been confirmed with other animals (mice, guinea pigs and monkeys). All species show the same effects.

Research published in the respected journal *Science* in the 1990s showed that calorie restriction in humans and other mammals switches on the anti-ageing genes: diet can effectively slow the ageing process (Lee et al., 1999). Further experiments have since shown that it's not only possible to slow the ageing process but also to reverse degenerative diseases associated with ageing (Cousens, 2005). It doesn't seem to matter at what age you begin to restrict calories in the diet, as within a short period of time after restricting sugar and starch, the ageing genes get switched off and youthing genes get switched on. There's real hope for those who want to live long, healthy lives. I have outlined details of a restricted calorie diet in my e-book, *The Big Fat Secret* (McKenna, 2012).

To date there is a massive volume of research showing the benefits of calorie restriction on blood pressure, heart disease, muscle strength, immunity, senile dementia, diabetes, raised

LDL cholesterol and autoimmune disorders (Cousens, 2005). This research confirms the negative role of too much carbohydrate in the Western diet and confirms why so many isolated cultures have thrived so well on little or no carbo-hydrates. Personally I have found that I have much more energy and feel a whole lot better when I abstain from or cut down on carbohydrates. Normally I only eat carbohydrate once a day at the main meal, but in winter I eat a lot more and I start to feel more sluggish. Carbohydrates such as starch (rice, pasta, potatoes, porridge, breads) are supposed to supply the body with glucose, which gives us energy, but too much taxes the liver and it gets overworked and sluggish. That's why a liver flush once a month is such a good idea. It's also why fasting is so helpful (more on that below).

Thomas Carn became famous in the UK in the Middle Ages, for reputedly living to be the ripe old age of 207. He was born in Shoreditch, London, in 1381 and according to the parish records, he died in 1588. His diet consisted of raw milk with butter and honey and some fruit for lunch and raw milk or fruit for supper with small amounts of bread occasionally; he did not eat breakfast. Despite such a severely restricted diet, he thrived.

So undereat rather than overeat. Don't wait for that feeling of fullness, but rather stop eating well before that. Follow the example of the Okinawans: eat little carbohydrate but eat vegetables and fish as often as you can.

Good food means little food. Good food means simple food. Good food means natural food.

FASTING

Fasting is one of the most amazing ways of helping your body to heal at all levels: physically, emotionally and spiritually. It literally lightens your body at an energy level by slowing your metabolic rate. You therefore need less energy to survive, in much the same way that you can slow your metabolism during meditation, deep relaxation and sleep and need little to sustain you.

I have experienced different types of fasting in my life, but the hardest by far was a soup fast that I did about 20 years ago. We were learning about the effects of fasting in theory by attending lectures for four hours in the morning and experiencing the effects physically by eating nothing other than a bowl of vegetable broth three times daily with as much water as we could drink. Every morning there were three litres of water outside my bedroom door, which I was supposed to drink during the day. I didn't manage to drink all three litres but tried to take what I could. I used to refer to the soup as the broth of life, as it was literally that.

I have never had a problem sleeping. Once I hit the pillow, I'm gone. However, doing this soup fast had a strong effect on me. I wasn't able to sleep at night and was pacing the floor at 2 a.m., trying to calm myself. My mind went into overdrive and I found it hard to stop the flow of thoughts. It was very hard to stop thinking about food. I was even hallucinating about food such as a big, juicy steak.

On the fourth day of the fast I refused the bowl of soup at 10 a.m. and was shocked to see myself push the bowl away. I thought I was going to be ravenous throughout the fast. It was quite a revelation that at different stages during the fast

I didn't feel hungry at all – quite the opposite, actually. I also felt much more energetic, both physically and mentally, and felt so much clearer in my thinking and much calmer emotionally overall. However, there were a few bad days when I felt nauseous and toxic. By the end of the second week my skin had cleared, I was full of energy and was full of the joys of life. This was the first time I had experienced fasting and soon realised it was an amazing healing tool for many complaints.

I had a German friend who was doing the fast too and he told me that he worked in a sanatorium where fasting was routinely used to treat a range of issues, from gynaecological problems to digestive complaints. For years he had treated patients by means of fasting but was now experiencing the benefits himself.

Basically, fasting lessens the workload on the liver. This is the organ responsible for getting toxic stuff out of the body and for creating energy for the body. It actually has many jobs and in my opinion is the most vital organ of them all. By fasting, you're giving your liver a chance to rest and repair itself. The liver has amazing powers of regeneration, so by giving it a chance to heal you're adding years to your life.

Fasting also helps the gut to rest and allows it to clear itself completely. There is often debris lodged on the wall of the gut, in much the same way that deposits form in your kettle or water pipes. Many health spas use herbs to cleanse the wall of the gut while fasting. Some health spas will use milk thistle or a mixture of herbs to assist the liver as well. They also use laxatives such as Epsom salts to ensure complete evacuation.

Fasting is a holiday for the principal parts of your body. You can do a three-day fast if you can't afford to take time off work.

You can begin on Friday morning and finish on Monday morning. If you can afford a little longer, you can do a five-day fast from Monday morning to Saturday morning, with the Sunday before as a preparation day and the Sunday after to phase back to a normal diet. For example, eat only fresh, raw foods such as fruit and salad on the Sunday before and after the fast. Then the fasting days are up to you. For example, you can do a fruit fast, a soup fast or a very strict water fast.

Fasting is best done in a group and under supervision. It's not recommended for those who are underweight (BMI of less than 18.5), those who are pregnant, breastfeeding, have diabetes or are on medication. You can do a fast at home, but make sure everyone knows what you're doing so that they can help you if you get into difficulty and support you if you break your fast. Fasting should really be done for at least seven days once a year and once a month for three days.

Recent research as shown on the BBC programme *The Power of Intermittent Fasting* (August 2012) shows that intermittent fasting has powerful health benefits as well. It involves fasting on alternate days. The fast that Dr Michael Mosley did wasn't really a fast at all in that he had eggs for breakfast, water and herbal teas throughout the day and fish and vegetables for dinner. He then ate normally the following day and then fasted the next day and so on for 21 days. There were marked improvements, as evidenced by blood tests done on him. I would recommend a stricter fast, such as soup only or fruit only on the fast days.

As you can see, fasting can be whatever you want it to be. The important point is to rest the liver and the gut for a period of time. Fasting not only has physical benefits, it also has a strong calming effect and lightens your body, thus increasing your awareness. I experienced this increased alertness and awareness very acutely towards the end of my strict two-week fast. My sensitivity increased to the point where I could taste ingredients in food that I couldn't taste before. I also found I could meditate much more easily and felt a profound sense of peace I had seldom felt. It was a great learning experience for me.

Fasting has a profound effect on your genetic make-up. I was taught to believe that your DNA or genetic make-up decides what health problems you will experience in life. We now know that this isn't the whole story. Nutrition plays a key role in switching certain genes on and others off. Food is the deciding factor in many illnesses. This is why fasting and restricted diets work so well in reversing so many illnesses. The science of how food influences your genes is called epigenetics. It's a fascinating field of study.

EPIGENETICS

I have a genetic predisposition to developing asthma, as many members of my family were asthmatic. I can remember my father having severe attacks when I was quite young and having to use an oxygen cylinder that was kept in his bedroom. I saw him suffer a lot with asthma and wanted to do everything possible to avoid the disease myself. I have never developed asthma and I attribute this to controlling my environment, especially what I eat. I was aware of this interplay of environment and genetic make-up from early on in my life.

Science is now showing that your genes (genome) or DNA is wrapped around proteins (histones) and both the DNA and the protein have receptors that receive messages all the time from the rest of the cell and from outside the cell. These messages or signals have the power to switch genes on or off. In other words, you may have inherited certain genes from your parents, but it's your environment that controls whether these genes will be switched on or off.

The receptors on the DNA and protein are called the epigenome. The major factor in determining whether I will or will not develop asthma is the epigenome, not the genome or DNA. The major environmental factor affecting the epigenome is your diet. This will play a significant role in determining which diseases you will get. Thus, environment, and particularly nutrition, plays a key role in both disease prevention and disease development. This is the opposite of what I was taught when I studied genetics many years ago, when it was believed that the genes or genome played the key role.

In the last 20 years, epigenetics has become very important in the field of science and medicine. It's now showing how all parts of the body are connected and how each cell is aware of what's happening outside the body in your environment. It's also showing how important diet and stress are in affecting or altering the epigenome. The epigenome is changing all the time in response to messages or signals. These messages or signals come from inside the cell, from cells close by and from your environment.

When a baby is developing in the womb, many of the signals come from the mother's body. It appears that the mother's diet and her stress levels have significant effects on the development of the baby's epigenome. The food that the mother eats is not only important for body building, but also for switching certain genes on and off. These genes will ultimately determine the anatomy (structure), physiology (function) and biochemistry (chemical reactions) of the baby. After birth, the external environment plays a bigger role in the child's epigenome. Again, the food given to the child, the level of stress in the family, physical exercise and, later, social interactions all play vital roles in the expression or non-expression of certain genes. Later still, hormonal changes will switch on the genes responsible for sexual maturity.

The epigenome is like an interface between your DNA and the environment. It's a dynamic structure in that it's constantly changing, in the same way that the messages received by your brain from your eyes, ears and other sense organs are causing changes in you all the time.

Epigenetics is showing that the body isn't a rigid structure, but is constantly in a state of flux and can adapt to almost anything. Your body is capable of much more than you believe possible. For instance, it's possible to delay and in certain cases reverse the ageing process. You are capable of living to over 200 years of age and you are capable of staying in good health for the duration of your life.

The key to healing and longevity is to know how to alter the diet in such a way that you can switch off the genes responsible for a disease and switch on the genes that will keep your body in good working order. Fasting works very well in this way for a whole range of disorders, and that is why many recommend it as a way of maintaining good health.

A patient who attended me many years ago had severe rheumatoid arthritis. She had tried almost every form of medicine and healing, all to no avail. We decided to use an exclusion diet with her for a two-week period and then reintro-duce other foods one at a time. The exclusion diet consisted of rice and lamb only, as these are the two least allergenic foods and so the least harmful. During the two-week period her pain level decreased gradually to the point where she was pain free for the first time in many years. She was so scared of the pain returning that she wanted to continue with the exclusion diet, so we extended it for another two weeks. As we reintroduced other foods one at a time, she started to react and resumed the exclusion diet of rice and lamb again for another month. It was very hard to convince her to continue with the reintroduction of other foods and eventually she gave up in frustration. Despite this, it was very revealing how diet had such a powerful effect on such a serious and debilitating disease.

Epigenetics is now showing how diet exerts its effects in the body. It's showing us that what happens in one part of the body has effects in all parts of the body. This may explain how reflexology, shiatsu, acupuncture and others forms of energetic healing can have such beneficial effects. Signals from the external environment travel to all cells of the body and affect the function of these cells via the epigenome. Ultimately, epigenetics will unite all forms of healing and will validate the key role of nutrition in medicine.

THE MAGIC IN FOOD

Food has a lot of magic attached to it. The basic elements that make up food are made in space. Water, which is the key prerequisite for life, has also come from space. In studying space, water and food, one is left reeling at how well life is orchestrated, down to the minutest chemical reaction. For example, water is the only known substance that has a lower density in its solid state. This is really ingenious, as it means that ice will therefore float on water, allowing fish to survive in winter. How clever is that? One is left in no doubt about the presence of a higher power.

For me, the most magical event of all is the conversion of sunlight into food. Green plants convert light particles from the sun into glucose. What's really strange and unusual about this process is that only a tiny amount of the energy is lost. Generally, at least 20 per cent of the energy is lost when energy is converted from one form to another in all reactions. In photosynthesis, however, over 99 per cent of the light energy is converted into chemical energy that forms the glucose molecule. There is clearly another process at work here.

The most unusual process I have learned about in the field of nutrition is the process called transmutation, a process whereby one element can change into a different element to facilitate the body. For example, seawater is known to contain very little calcium (about 0.04 per cent). This is far too little for shellfish to be able to make shells, which are composed of calcium carbonate. So where does all the calcium come from to make these shells? The bodies of some of these animals were analysed and it was discovered that the body also has too little calcium. Clearly, these animals can produce calcium from another element.

In his research in the Sahara Desert, Dr Kervan discovered that the workers ate an excess of salt in their diet and excreted far more potassium than they consumed. Where was all the potassium coming from? He postulated that it was the result of an endothermic reaction (uses up heat) and so it had a cooling effect. The endothermic reaction was the combination of sodium (salt) and oxygen to form potassium. In his book *Biological Transmutations* (1972), he suggests this is yet another example of transmutation. Today there are a number of examples of biological transmutation, yet orthodox science refuses to accept it, as it contradicts the laws of physics.

Another amazing finding is the incredibly important role bacteria play in the lives of all living creatures. Soil bacteria serve the needs of plants by making nitrogen compound for them. We are colonised by trillions of bacteria, which serve many vital functions in our body. They do so much for us that life without them would be impossible. They may be microscopic single-celled organisms, but we owe our lives to them. These simple cells have the ability to outsmart us humans by rendering many of our antibiotics useless – they can develop resistant genes in the space of a few generations. There is clearly a much higher intelligence at work here.

And so the magic goes on as long as we trust and stay close to Nature and to our own true nature. Don't heed advice from outside, as the real intelligence and wisdom reside within you. The authorities are sadly lacking in both intelligence and wisdom. As the world changes dramatically, increase your self-reliance and don't be dependent on the authorities for anything.

Chapter 9
Conclusion

The time for simple, wholesome food has returned. I can see a huge demand for real food in the years ahead, when supermarkets will be forced to change, farmers will abandon chemically treated crops for traditional methods and parents will have more time to enjoy the art of preparing food at home with their families. The time for processed food has passed; its days are numbered. People are waking up to many hard truths about all aspects of life and are becoming aware that one does not have to live a life being a slave to the system: to mortgage repayments, to the banks, to a particular religious belief. The internet is part of this revolution. It has only taken off in the last two decades and has had an amazing effect on people's lives, destroying old belief systems and connecting people in incredible ways. Amidst this revolution is a growing demand for simple, healthy food and water. The structures in our society will have to satisfy that demand.

People in the UK, US and Ireland have steadily increased in body weight over the past three decades, to the point where there are fewer and fewer men and women of normal weight. This is down to the changes in foodstuffs manufactured by food processors in the US and UK. These companies have destroyed the natural balances in the body and put toxic substances into the food chain. This began in the mid-1970s with the addition of high fructose corn syrup and in the 1980s with the addition of artificial sweeteners. These two additions have damaged more humans on this planet than any other substances in the history of mankind.

The work of Dr Weston Price in the 1930s forewarned about the dangers of processed foods, especially those with white flour and sugar. He showed the negative effects of these foods not only on the teeth, but on general health and physical vitality. The research of Professor John Yudkin warned of the dangers of too much fructose in the diet and essentially described the obesity epidemic we are presently living with.

We have been misinformed and deliberately lied to about the role of animal fat in the diet. This lie has been reinforced with the introduction of a food pyramid and later, a food plate. The Food Safety Authority (and the Food and Drug Administration in the US) have discredited themselves for allowing items into the food chain that have been proven to cause cancers in animals and in humans. Pharmaceutical companies have allowed some of these dangerous chemicals into common medicines and vitamin tablets for adults and children. The medical profession and the dieticians have stayed strangely silent and in turn have discredited themselves as well.

The control that chemical companies such as Monsanto have over farmers is about to change. The revolving door between Monsanto and the US Administration will have to shut and politicians will have to be seen to be free from vested interests. Too many officials advising the US government are or have been employees of Monsanto, the most prominent being Donald Rumsfeld. The legislation that gives this company the right to vet independent research on their genetically modified seeds has to be abolished. Farmers must be free to farm and not be servants of the food industry. Consumers must be vigilant and exert pressure on the supermarkets to sell fresh produce and remove harmful processed foods.

The production and selling of food is the biggest industry in the world. You are a part of that industry. If you don't like what's happening, do something about it. Start by supporting those farmers who offer healthy produce for sale in farmers' markets and farm shops. For the sake of your family, your global family and the planet you presently reside on, demand good food.

The planet you live on is a living structure providing you with all the food you need. It's likened to your mother, who collects this food, prepares it and cooks it to help you stay healthy. The planet is here to serve you, to provide you with all you need. It's an essential link in the chain connecting you with creation. It's regarded as sacred by all primitive peoples.

If you truly appreciate this fact, you will realise quite quickly that it is in nobody's best interest to pollute it, poison it, destroy its atmosphere or dig big holes in its surface. Every time you drive your car, you're supporting the oil industry that gouges holes in the planet, pollutes vast areas with oil spills and poisons the atmosphere with exhaust fumes. Every time you take a flight, which is regarded as routine these days, you are again supporting the destruction of Earth. Your culture regards this as progress, as a step forward in our scientific understanding, as a magical means of travel. If you poison your parent or dig holes in their bodies or pollute the air they breathe, is that called progress? Is that called scientific advancement? No. It's called murder. By blindly or overtly co-operating with this murder of our planet, you and I become an accomplice. We are as guilty as the oil companies, the food companies, the chemical companies and the pharmaceutical companies.

It simply makes no sense at any level to poison the being that feeds you. It's self-destructive to do so. However, that is how we live our lives, especially in the West. We are so arrogant and proud that we can't see the truth of our actions. We have been so blinded by our scientific advancements that we can't see the big picture. It's a scientific advancement to be able to convert nitrogen in the air into organic nitrogen (ammonia), as Fritz Haber did in the early 1900s, but it's self-destructive to use this ammonia on soil if it weakens the plants and requires frequent doses of chemical sprays to keep the plants alive, especially if these chemicals end up in the food chain and cause a myriad of health problems. Virtually everyone practising natural medicine tells people to avoid wheat or in some cases all gluten cereals (wheat, rye, oats and barley), as they are causing so many health problems. These cereals are among the most polluted on the planet.

If you truly believe Earth is a living structure, then you must know it will heal itself, but perhaps at great expense to us. Nature will right itself, but in its own way and its own good time. Heal your own true nature and don't allow fear to control your actions. Base your actions on love: love of yourself, love of other beings and love of the planet you live on. If you're kind to yourself, you're more likely to be kind to others and to respect the planet. Then your eyes will open to the self-destructive nature of our society and to the nature of the foods we feed ourselves.

You have the choice to continue to behave as if everything is okay and lead your life as you are now and support all the structures that make up Western society. By doing so, you're putting your faith and energy in Western society and so encouraging it to grow and expand. Or you can start to change your ways: the way you shop, the way you prepare food, the way you consume energy, the way you educate your children, the way you watch television, and so on.

If you wish to change, then start with food, as this is the cornerstone of your life. By thinking about food and making good choices, you will learn not just about nutrition, but about the whole of your society. Many people over the years that I saw in practice have echoed the sentiment that they learned so much simply by changing their diets. It's true, as it forces you to think about everything you put in your mouth; what was a subconscious process becomes a much more conscious decision. You slowly gain control over your eating habits.

If you wish to change, then start today. Begin by eliminating all sugar from your diet and your body will function much better. Then eliminate all food additives, especially artificial sweeteners. By doing this you are essentially eliminating all processed foods, which is a major step forward towards a healthier diet. Then avoid all non-organic dairy and if possible use raw milk. Finally, eliminate wheat and all wheat products – use spelt bread instead.

By supporting a healthy diet for you and your loved ones, you are making the planet a better place for all of us, as your choices will influence farmers, supermarkets and ultimately all food producers in our society.

Thank you for taking the time to read this book.

Bibliography

Abou-Donia, M.B. et al., 'Splenda alters gut microflora and increases intestinal P-glycoprotein and cytochrome P450 in male rats', *Journal of Toxicology and Environmental Health*, Part A, 71/21 (2008), 1,415–29.

Ahrens, E.H., 'Carbohydrates, plasma triglycerides and coronary heart disease', *Nutrition Reviews*, 44/2 (1986), 60–4.

Boik, J., *Natural Compound in Cancer Therapy*, Princeton, MN: Oregon Medical Press, 2001.

Campbell, C. and Campbell, T., *The China Study: The Most Comprehensive Study of Nutrition Ever Conducted and the Startling Implications for Diet, Weight Loss, and Long-term Health*, Dallas: Benbella Books Inc., 2006.

Chandra, R.K., 'Excessive intake of zinc impairs immune response', *Journal of the American Medical Association*, 252 (1984), 1,443–6.

Cousens, G., *Spiritual Nutrition*, Berkley: North Atlantic Books, 2005.

Daley, C.A., 'A review of fatty acid profiles in grass-fed and grain-fed beef', *Nutrition Journal*, 9 (2010), 10.

Davies, S. and Stewart, A., *Nutritional Medicine*, London: Pan Macmillan, 1987.

De Luca, L.M., 'Retinoids in differentiation and neoplasia', *Scientific American Science and Medicine* (July–August 1995), 28–36.

Epstein, S., *The Politics of Cancer Revisited*, Fremont, NY: East Ridge Press, 1998.

Fallon, S., *Nourishing Traditions*, Washington: New Trends Pub Inc., 2001.

Gaskell, K., *Green Tea: The Latest Research on Its Proposed Health Benefits*, Amazon Kindle, 2013.

Hamilton, G., 'Insider trading', *New Scientist* (26 June 1999), 43–5.

Harrill, R., *Using a Refractometer to Test the Quality of Fruits and Vegetables*, Redlands: Pine Knoll Publications, 1994.

Harvey, G., *We Want Real Food*, London: Robinson, 2008.

Hungerford, C., *The Good Body Guide*, London: Marion Boyars, 2009.

Jacobsen, M., Lefferts, L. and Garland, A., *Safe Food*, New York: Berkley, 1993.

Johnson, R.J. et al., 'Potential role of sugar (fructose) in the epidemic of hypertension, obesity and the metabolic syndrome, diabetes, kidney disease and cardiovascular disease', *American Journal of Clinical Nutrition*, 86/4 (October 2007), 899–906.

Kendrick, M., *The Great Cholesterol Con*, London: John Blake Publishers, 2007.

Kervan, C.L., *Biological Transmutations*, New York: Swan House Publishing Co., 1972.

Keys, A., 'Coronary heart disease in seven countries', *Circulation*, 41 (supplement) (1970), 1–211.

Keys, A. et al., 'Inter-cohort differences in coronary heart disease mortality in the 25-year follow-up to the seven countries study', *European Journal of Epidemiology*, 9/5 (September 1993), 527–36.

Lee, C-K., Klopp, R., Weindruch, R. and Prolla, T., 'Gene expression profile of ageing and its retardation by caloric restriction', *Science* (27 August 1999), 1,390–3.

Lopez, A., 'Some interesting relationships between dietary carbohydrate and serum cholesterol', *American Journal of Clinical Nutrition*, 18 (1966), 149–53.

Mann, G.V. et al., 'Atherosclerosis in the Masai', *American Journal of Epidemiology*, 95/1 (January 1972), 26–37.

McKenna, J., *Natural Alternatives to Antibiotics*, Dublin: Gill & Macmillan, 1996.

McKenna, J., *Hard to Stomach: Real Solutions to Your Digestive Problems*, Dublin: New Leaf, 2002.

McKenna, J., *The Big Fat Secret*, London: Jemsoil Publishers, Amazon Kindle, 2012.

O'Doherty, C., '30,000 homes at risk of lead poisoning from water', *Irish Examiner*, 3 January 2013.

Ontario College of Family Physicians, *Review of Research on Effects of Pesticides on Human Health*, 2012. Available at www.ocfp.on.ca.

Oski, F., *Don't Drink Your Milk*, Ringold: TEACH Services Inc., 1992.

Oster, K., 'Plasmalogen: a new concept of the etiology of the atherosclerotic process', *American Journal of Clinical Research*, 2 (1971), 30–5.

Oster, K. and Ross, D., 'The presence of ectopic xanthine oxidase in atherosclerotic plagues and myocardial tissue', *Proceedings of the Society for Experimental Biology and Medicine* (1973).

Oster, K., Oster, J. and Ross, D., 'Immune response to bovine xanthine oxidase in atherosclerotic patients', *American*

Laboratory (August 1974), 41–7.

Pottenger, F.M., *Pottenger's Cats: A Study in Nutrition*, California: Price-Pottenger Nutrition Foundation, 1995.

Price, W.A., *Nutrition and Physical Degeneration*, California: Price-Pottenger Nutrition Foundation, 2008.

Qin, K. et al., 'What made Canada become a country with the highest incidence of IBD: Could sucralose be the culprit?', *Canadian Journal of Gastroenterology*, 25/9 (2011), 511.

Qin, K. et al., 'Etiology of IBD: A unified hypothesis', *World Journal of Gastroenterology*, 18/15 (2012), 1,708–22.

Schernhammer, E. et al., 'Consumption of artificial sweetener and sugar-containing soda and risk of lymphoma and leukaemia in men and women', *American Journal of Clinical Nutrition*, 96 (2012), 1,419–28.

Shankar, A.H., 'The effect of vitamin A supplementation on morbidity due to plasmodium falciparum in young children in Papua New Guinea: A randomised trial', *The Lancet*, 354 (17 July 1999), 302–9.

Shils, M.E. et al., *Modern Nutrition in Health and Disease*, Philadelphia: Lea & Febiger, 1994.

Soffritti, M. et al., 'Life span exposure to low doses of aspartame beginning during prenatal life increases cancer effects in rats', *Environmental Health Perspectives*, 115 (2007), 1,293–7.

Stoddard, M.N., *Deadly Deception: The Story of Aspartame*, Dallas: Oderwald Press, 1998.

Tsubono, Y., 'Plasma antioxidant vitamins and carotenoids in five Japanese populations with varied mortality from gastric cancer', *Nutrition and Cancer*, 34/1 (1999), 56–61.

University of Maryland Medical Center, 'Green tea',
    available online at www.umm.edu/altmed/articles/green-
    tea-000255.htm.
Whetsell, W., 'Current concepts of excitotoxicity', *Journal of
    Neuropathology and Experimental Neurology*, 55 (1996),
    1,115–23.
Yudkin, J., *Pure, White and Deadly* (new edition), London:
    Penguin, 2012.

Resources

SUPPLIERS OF GOOD WATER

Isklar, Sabco Group, PO 3779, Postal Code 112, Ruwi,
Sultanate of Oman. www.sabcogroup.com.
Tel. 968 2466 0100. E-mail info@sabcogroup.com

Spa, Brecon Water, Trap, near Llandeilo, Carmarthenshire,
Wales SA19, 67T. www.breconwater.co.uk.
Tel. 44 1269 850175. E-mail sales@breconwater.co.uk

Pellegrino S.p.A., via Lodovico Il Moro 35, 20143 Milan, Italy.
www.sanpellegrino.com

SUPPLIERS OF GOOD PROBIOTICS

Optibac Probiotics, 15 Towergate Business Park, Colebrook
Way, Andover, Hampshire SP10 3BB.
www.optibacprobiotics.co.uk. Tel. 44 1264 339770.
E-mail sales@mediapharma.co.uk

Biocare Ltd, Lakeside, 180 Lifford Lane, Kings Norton,
Birmingham B30 3NU. www.biocare.co.uk.
Tel. 44 121 433 3727. E-mail customerservice@biocare.co.uk

SUPPLIERS OF GOOD FAT AND PROTEIN

Laverstoke Farm – UK. North Overton, Overton, Hampshire
RG25 3DR. www.laverstokepark.co.uk. Tel. 0800 394 5505

Ballymore Farm – Ireland. E-mail www.ballymorefarm.ie

SUPPLIERS OF FLAXSEED OIL

Virginia Harvest, Virginia Health Food Ltd, Oysterhaven,
Kinsale, Co. Cork. www.virginiafoods.net. Tel. 353 21 4790033.
E-mail info@virginiafoods.net

Udo's Choice, www.udoschoice.ie. Tel. 353 404 82444.
E-mail customerservices@udochoice.ie

SUPPLIERS OF VITAMINS AND MINERALS

Solgar, Beggars Lane, Aldbury, Tring, Herts HP23 5PT.
www.solgar.com/uk. Tel. 44 1442 89055.
E-mail solgarinfo@solgar.com

Biocare Ltd, Lakeside, 180 Lifford Lane, Kings Norton,
Birmingham B30 3NU. www.biocare.co.uk.
Tel. 44 121 433 3727. E-mail customerservice@biocare.co.uk

SUPPLIERS OF GREEN TEA

High Teas, www.highteas.co.uk

Index

Page numbers in **bold** refer to diagrams in the text.

American Dietetic Association,
   sponsorship of food companies 45–6
American Heart Association 32, 39
American Journal of Clinical Nutrition
   140
American Journal of Epidemiology 41
American National Toxicology
   Program 115
amino acids 30, 92, 93, 138, 151
ammonia 120, 121, 122, 185
Amoxil 142
animal fat *see* saturated fats
animals *see* livestock
antibiotics 85, 181
   aspartame in 142
   in milk 133
   resistance to 133
antibodies 70
anticarcinogens 71, 108, 130, 131
antioxidants
   cholesterol as 48
   vitamin A 108
   vitamins as 106–7
anxiety 144
appendix operations 22
artesian wells 80, 115
arthritis 8
   incidence in Africa/traditional diet x
   osteoarthritis 19, 23, 38, 71
   rheumatoid 72, 178–9
   and vegetables 148
   and Western diet x
artificial fertilisers 121–4
   and crops 123
   damage to lakes and rivers 123, 124
   and microbial content of soil 124
   water table pollution 123
artificial sweeteners 85, 114, 118, 126,
   136–42
   and brain tumours 136–7
   exclude from diet 186
   and headaches 139
   reactions to taking 144
   research studies on 140–41, 142–3
   sucralose 142–5
   tumours in experimental animals 144
aspartame 114, 118, 146
   development of 137–8
   in diet drinks 137

and diketopiperazine (DKP) 138
and formaldehyde 138–9
and headaches 139
in medicines 137
   medicines containing 141–2
and tumours 137, 138, 141
in vitamin tablets 137, 141
asthma 8, 19, 126, 176
aubergine 8
Augmentin 142
autism 126
auto-immune disorders 72, 172
avocados 90, 111
Ayrshire cows 160

babies *see* infants
bacon, organic 151
bacteria
   and B vitamins 83
   bad bacteria in the gut 67
   and body composition 62, 82, 181
   coating on all surfaces of the body 83
   good bacteria 82–5, 150
   good bacteria in raw milk 62
   gut bacteria 83–5
   lactic acid-producing bacteria 62, 82
   micronutrients and gut flora 83
   probiotic cultures 82
   in soil 163, 181
   and sugar 67
bacterial flora 83–5, 142, 143
'bad' cholesterol *see* LDL (low-density
   lipoprotein)
Ballymore Farm 160
bananas 111
barley 20, 152, 185
BASF 120, 121
bear 23
beef 54, 73, 151
beer 152
Benadryl 142
bentonite clay 101, 105
berries 21, 38
beta carotene 108
BHA *see* butylated hydroxyanisole
BHT *see* butylated hydroxytoluene
bifidobacterium 143
Big Fat Secret, The (McKenna) 57, 98,
   117, 171